AMERICAN JOURNAL of PUBLIC HEALTH
AUGUST 2023
Issue 8

AJPH

A PUBLICATION OF THE
AMERICAN PUBLIC HEALTH ASSOCIATION

TOBACCO DEPENDENCE IN CURRENTLY SMOKING ADOLESCENTS WORLDWIDE

What Lies Ahead?, p. 859
Commercial Determinants, p. 856
Prevalence and Risk Factors, p. 861

Also in this issue:

SOGI DATA
In US Health Centers, pp. 834 and 883

COVID-19
High-Throughput Vaccination Sites, pp. 836 and 909

US IMMIGRANT HOUSECLEANERS
Impact of COVID-19, p. 893

PUBLIC HEALTH CRISPR
Health Equity Issues, p. 874

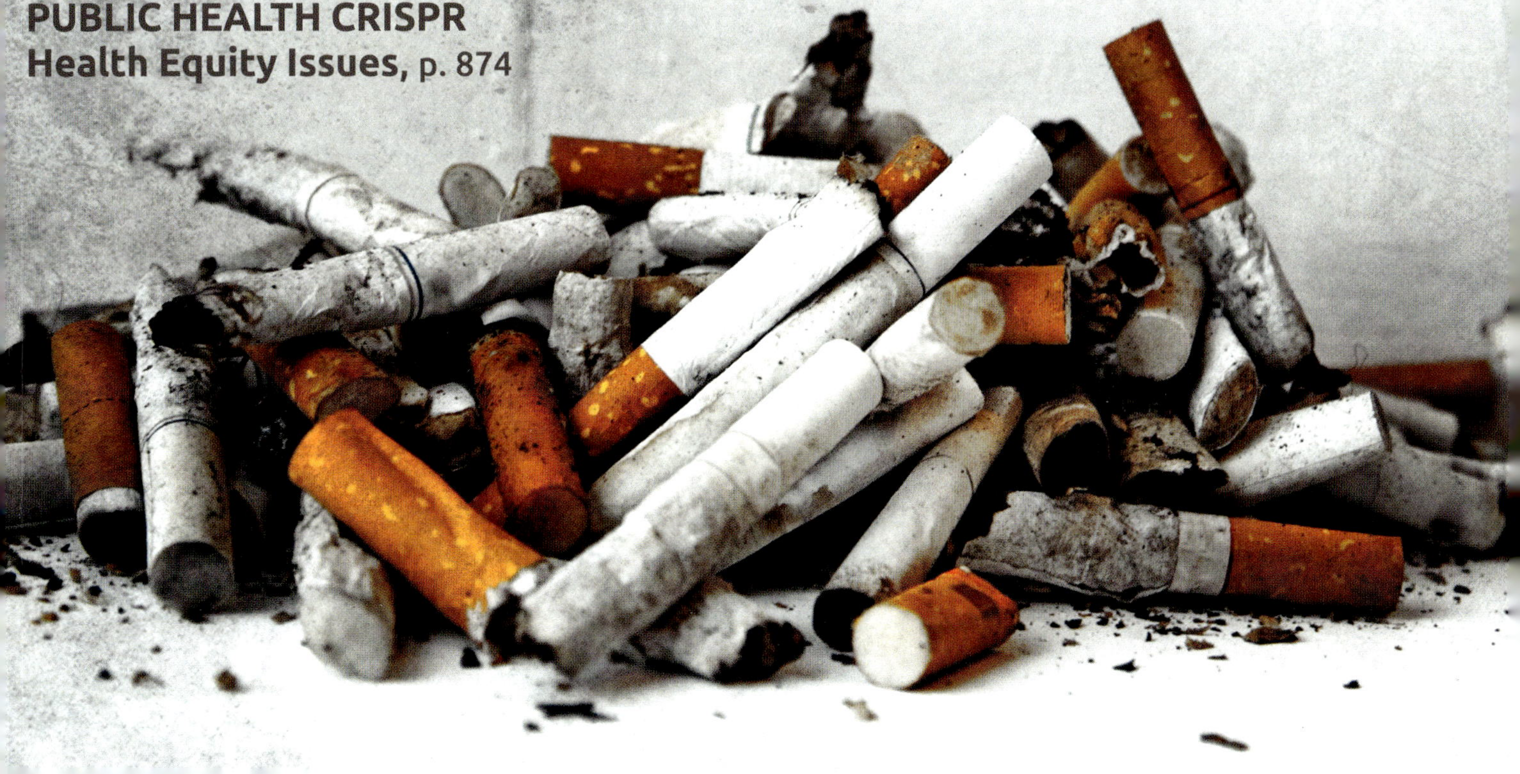

APHA
AMERICAN PUBLIC HEALTH ASSOCIATION
For science. For action. For health.

AJPH®, published monthly, is the official Journal of the American Public Health Association®, 800 I St NW, Washington, DC 20001-3710; (202) 777- APHA; TDD (202) 777-2500. APHA is a nongovernmental professional society founded in 1872, representing all disciplines and specialties in public health.

The *American Journal of Public Health*® (*AJPH*) (print ISSN: 0090-0036; electronic ISSN: 1541- 0048), first published in 1911, is the official journal of the American Public Health Association® (APHA). The oldest and largest organization of public health professionals in the world, APHA represents approximately 30 000 members from more than 50 occupations of public health.

Submissions: Visit www.editorialmanager.com/ajph or ajph.edmgr.com for online manuscript preparation and submission guidelines. Contributions of original unpublished research, social science analyses, scholarly essays, critical commentaries, departments, and letters to the editor are welcome. Questions? Write ajph.submissions@apha.org or call APHA at (202) 777-2469.

Print plus online subscriptions: Institutional price (print copy with online access for a single institution and all authorized users, regardless of geographic location) varies by size of organization and ranges from $993–$1445 for US organizations, and $1073–$1526 for international organizations (air delivery); multiple campuses not permitted without special arrangement. Details of the tiered pricing system at https://subscriptionoffice.com/pages/apha-landing-page. To order, write apha.subscriptions@apha.org.

Online-only subscriptions: Institutional price for one institution and its authorized users (regardless of geographic location) is $878–$1307. To order, write apha.subscriptions@apha.org. For academic consortia or multisite corporate subscriptions, contact apha.subscriptions@apha.org.

Print-only subscriptions: Institutional price is US $701, $782 international.

Back print issues: A limited number of print issues are for sale. Single copies are US $49, $55 international (air delivery). Shipping included; prepay only. To order, write apha.subscriptions@apha.org.

Reprints: For prices and ordering information on 50 or more reprints, check the Reprints section at www.ajph.org. To order smaller quantities of reprints (rush delivery), use the "Purchase Article" link on the article site itself.

Electronic access: Online articles more than 10 years old are available free for personal use at www.ajph.org. Recent articles are available through pay-per-view: single PDF article for $24, single issue access for 24 hours for $33, or entire site access for 24 hours for $38.

Postal information: Periodicals postage paid at Washington, DC, and additional mailing offices. Postmaster: Send address changes to American Journal of Public Health, 800 I St NW, Washington, DC 20001-3710.

Address changes: Send to AJPH, Membership Department (members) or AJPH Subscriptions (subscribers), APHA, 800 I St NW, Washington, DC 20001-3710. Or write to membership.mail@apha. org (members) or apha.subscriptions@apha.org (subscribers).

Advertising: For pricing and other information, see www.ajph.org. Please write to ashell.alston@apha.org or call (202) 777-2470 for other advertising opportunities. Ask about special exhibit packages and sponsorships. Acceptance of advertising by the *Journal* does not imply endorsement of products.

Indexes: Publications that index or abstract articles from AJPH include the following: Ageline, Assia (Applied Social Science Index and Abstracts), Biological Abstracts, Chemical Abstracts, CINAHL, Criminal Justice Abstracts, EMBASE, EMCare, Environmental Abstracts, e-psyche, ERIC, ETOH (Alcohol and Alcohol Problems Science Database), Excerpta Medica, Food Science and Technology, General Science Index, Grateful Med, Hospital Literature Index, Human Resources Abstracts, International Pharmaceutical Abstracts (IPA), Medline, Physical Education Index, Pollution Abstracts, Psychological Abstracts, PsychINFO, Safety Science Abstracts, Sage Family Studies Abstracts, Sage Human Resources Abstracts, Science Citation Index, SCOPUS, SIIC Data Bases, Social Work Research and Abstracts, and Statistical Reference Index (SRI)/LexisNexis.

Medscape Publishers' Circle

AJPH

A PUBLICATION OF THE
AMERICAN PUBLIC HEALTH ASSOCIATION

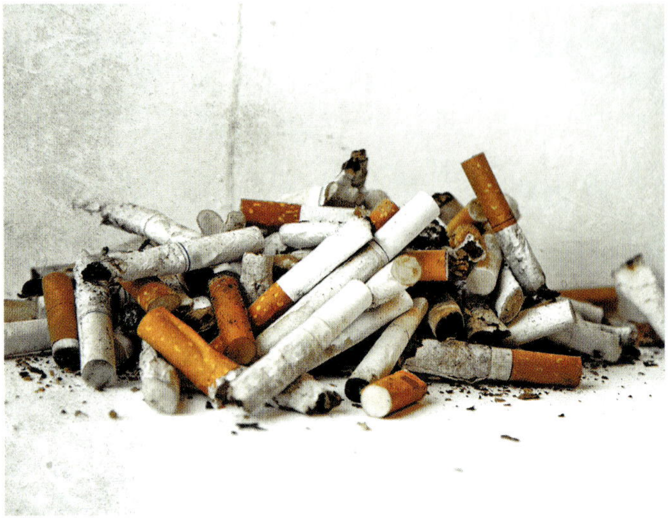

COVER: Nearly 40% of adolescents who are currently smoking tobacco report tobacco dependence. Smoking cessation and health education programs should consider trends in the prevalence of tobacco dependence among adolescents.

Cover concept and selection by Aleisha Kropf. Photo by Marlene Ford/Getty Images. Printed with permission.

APHA
AMERICAN PUBLIC HEALTH ASSOCIATION
For science. For action. For health.

Promoting public health research, policy, practice, and education is the *AJPH* mission. As we widen our scope to embrace global issues, we also sharpen our focus to support the needs of public health practitioners. We invite contributions of original unpublished research, opinion and commentary, and letters to the editor.

The *Journal* is printed on acid-free recycled paper.

AJPH August 2023, Vol 113, No. 8

OPEN ACCESS · ONLINE ONLY · PODCAST · DATA SUPPLEMENT AVAILABLE

EDITOR'S CHOICE

828 Absurdities About COVID-19 and Public Health
A. Morabia

BOOKS & MEDIA

829 How Three Clinical Professions Addressed Disability in Recent Decades
D. Fox and J. M. Perrin

832 Winning Rights: The Role of Worker Centers in Protecting the Most Vulnerable Workers
M. Goldstein-Gelb and L. S. Marin

OPINIONS, IDEAS, & PRACTICE

EDITORIALS

834 Improvements in Sexual Orientation and Gender Identity Data Collection Through Policy and Education
M. Stasenko and G. P. Quinn

836 Vaccinating the Masses During a Pandemic: Learning in Real Time for Tomorrow
H. M. Brandt

839 Data Democratization for Health Equity: A Public Health of Consequence, August 2023
F. Kapadia

PERSPECTIVES

841 East Palestine, Ohio, Railroad Derailment—Lessons to Learn, Actions to Take
C. M. Schooling, H. E. Jones, and S. McDermott

844 Where Was Climate Change at the White House Conference on Hunger, Nutrition, and Health?
R. G. Clark, S. Pryor, and W. H. Dietz

849 Improving Indian Health Service Vaccination Campaigns Across the Full Spectrum of Age, Clinical, and Public Health Settings
H. A. Baker, A. Klunk, A. J. Calac, T. Livermont, and S. Bell

852 Why Are We Going Backward? Barriers to Disaggregated Racial Information in Federal Data Sets
A. Jamal, M. Srinivasan, G. Kim, R. J. Huang, and L. Palaniappan

TOBACCO DEPENDENCE AMONG ADOLESCENTS

856 Addressing Commercial Determinants to End High Tobacco Dependence Among Adolescents
A. Peruga and E. Fernández

859 Tobacco Dependence in Adolescents: What Lies Ahead?
R. Mehrotra, K. Yadav, and K. Siddiqi

RESEARCH & ANALYSIS

TOBACCO DEPENDENCE AMONG ADOLESCENTS

861 Prevalence of and Factors Associated With Tobacco Dependence Among Adolescents Aged 12–16 Years Who Were Currently Smoking Tobacco in 125 Countries or Territories, 2012–2019
H. Yang, C. Ma, M. Zhao, and B. Xi

OPEN-THEMED RESEARCH

870 The Pent-Up Demand for Breastfeeding Among US Women: Trends After COVID-19 Shelter-in-Place
R. Hamad, D. F. Collin, A. Gemmill, K. Jackson, and D. Karasek

874 CRISPR in Public Health: The Health Equity Implications and Role of Community in Gene-Editing Research and Applications
A. M. Subica

883 Sexual Orientation and Gender Identity Data Completeness at US Federally Qualified Health Centers, 2020 and 2021
M. Liu, D. King, K. H. Mayer, C. Grasso, and A. S. Keuroghlian

893 COVID-19 Infections, Pandemic-Related Social and Economic Impacts, and Changes to Mental and Self-Rated Health Among Latinx Immigrant Housecleaners in New York City: The Safe and Just Cleaners Study
S. Baron, I. Cuervo, D. Shah, A. Gonzalez, H. Harari, and D. Flores

904 SARS-CoV-2 Cases Reported on International Arriving and Domestic Flights: United States, January 2020–December 2021
L. E. Preston, A. Rey, S. Dumas, A. Rodriguez, A. M. Gertz, K. C. Delea, F. Alvarado-Ramy, D. L. Christensen, C. Brown, and T.-H. Chen

909 Promising Practices Observed in High-Throughput COVID-19 Vaccination Sites in the United States, February–May 2021
C. E. McColloch, M. E. Samson, K. Anne Parris, A. Stewart, J. A. Robinson, B. Cooper, E. Galloway, R. Garcia, Z. Gilani, B. Jayapaul-Philip, P. Lucas, K. H. Nguyen, R. S. Noe, A.-R. T. Trudeau, and E. D. Kennedy

BACKMATTER

ERRATA

919 Erratum In: "'Ashamed to Put My Name to It': Monsanto, Industrial Bio-Test Laboratories, and the Use of Fraudulent Science, 1969–1985"

OTHER DEPARTMENTS

928 Subscription Form

Absurdities About COVID-19 and Public Health

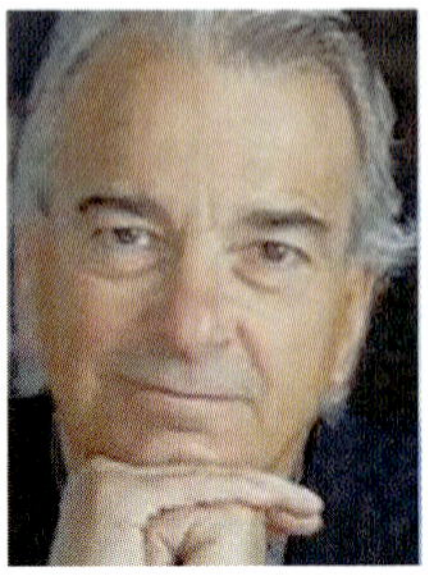

Some attempts to belittle the role of public health in the response to the COVID-19 pandemic are simply absurd. There is no doubt that vaccine coverage saved lives. The proportion of physicians per capita (https://bit.ly/3IXjHVs) was not associated with greater vaccine coverage in red states (https://bit.ly/3NguBbF). The vaccine worked, and doctors per capita doesn't explain the differences in full vaccine coverage, which in red states ranges from about 50% (Alabama) to 70% (Florida). How, then, could the vaccines have gone successfully from the warehouses of the pharmaceutical industry into the arms of millions of Americans if it were not because of public health?

The reality is that, despite its chronic underfunding, the public health response to COVID-19 has been an achievement that stands out in the history of US public health. As Michael Fraser and Brent Ewig put it in their indispensable book, *Vaccinating America: The Inside Story Behind the Race to Save Lives, and End a Pandemic* (Washington, DC: APHA Press; 2022), "Never in American history had so many vaccines been delivered and administered in such a short time" (pp. 108–109). Almost 200 million doses in three months. Consider also the proportion of persons aged 65 years and older fully vaccinated against COVID-19. It is a landslide. On average, 93% of the population was vaccinated; 24 states vaccinated almost all their seniors. The worst achiever, Arkansas, vaccinated 83% of them. Public health was effective and saved lives throughout the country. Public health agencies rose to the challenge even in the states where the greatest opposition was mobilized against it.

To assess the real role of public health during the crisis, knowledge of the process that turned "vaccines into vaccinations," as Fraser and Ewig write, is essential. Tens of thousands of provider sites had to be enrolled and trained to properly store, handle, and administer the vaccine in accordance with Centers for Disease Control and Prevention (CDC) recommendations, to order ancillary supplies, and to report on administrations and possible side effects.

It is important to note that statistics about health care workers per capita, public health employees per capita, and public health spending per capita cannot reflect the full role of public health. For example, 43% of all COVID-19 vaccine doses were administered through partnership between the public health and pharmacies (p. 118). The CDC's Pharmacy Partnership for Long Term Health Program was aimed at nursing homes, while the Federal Retail Pharmacy Program relied on public health agencies encouraging individuals to go to pharmacies. Millions of Americans, however, have no access to pharmacies, so governmental public health departments had to set up vaccination clinics, including mobile clinics, to meet local demand. Governmental public health departments had to perform vaccinations that no one else wanted to do, as well as work with community-based organizations and at their own clinical sites.

The response to COVID-19 could have saved even more lives. This was within the reach of public health had it not been hampered by errors committed by the leaders of Operation Warp Speed, such as side-lining the CDC in favor of personnel inexperienced in public health (https://bit.ly/45KSKhv), slow engagement, and insufficient funding of state and local public health agencies (*Vaccinating America*, pp. 53-54).

There are several additional limitations of the available data and their interpretation that warrant caution when attempting to quantify the specific impact of public health in the response. In particular:

1. We don't know what the infection rate from SARS-CoV-2 (the causative agent of COVID-19) has been because there has not been a federal population-based survey similar to ENE-COVID in Spain (https://bit.ly/3WTuwNX) or REACT-1 in the United Kingdom (https://bit.ly/3MQ5lax). For example, rates of asymptomatic infections are not known.
2. COVID-19 deaths have been tagged differently across institutions and across the country, overrepresented in some cases, underrepresented in others (https://bit.ly/3qoO8xr). It is not a highly accurate outcome.
3. Excess deaths during the pandemic, compared with the number of deaths expected on the basis of prepandemic years, are the best proxy for the impact of COVID-19.
4. States are not a good unit of analysis for the impact of COVID-19. They are too heterogeneous. For example, take Texas. Houston, Austin, and Dallas had high vaccine coverage, whereas the rural countryside did not. Look at a Google map of King County (https://bit.ly/3WRoVI2), which had one of the lowest vaccine coverages in the state. When the GPS says you have arrived in Guthrie, the county seat, on US Route 82, you can only see prairie for miles on a 360° view—not a single building. Comparing counties across the United States should provide fairer comparisons than state-level ones.

The paucity of health-monitoring data is a huge component of the alleged poor performance of the United States in the COVID-19 pandemic. Unfortunately, absurd statements belittling the key role of public health in the overall response will continue to be produced and reproduced ad nauseam by those who have made public health their target. AJPH

Alfredo Morabia, MD, PhD
Editor-in-Chief, AJPH

DOI: https://doi.org/10.2105/AJPH.2023.307357

33 Years Ago

Tobacco Taxation as Health Policy in the Third World

The worldwide mortality toll of tobacco—already a pandemic of 2.5 million deaths each year—is projected by the World Health Organization to rise five-fold to 12 million by the middle of the next century, with most of the increase occurring in the [less developed countries]. . . . The brown plague is metastasizing to the Third World. The level of ignorance in these countries about the effects of tobacco is profound. The marketing tactics of the transnational tobacco companies are astonishingly aggressive, devoid of even the pretense of civility in which developed country marketers attempt to cloak their advertising and promotion. Strong antitobacco health policies are desperately needed, but the prospects are limited. In such an environment, encouraging governments to increase tobacco taxes to promote health will be a daunting task. But it is one well worth pursuing.

From AJPH, *May 1990, pp. 529–530.*

54 Years Ago

Health Needs of Adolescents: How the Adolescent Sees Them

The study of health problems, as seen by adolescents themselves, has not received attention in any systematic fashion. How do adolescents view their own health? What do they see as major health problems for themselves and their contemporaries? What is the significance of their attitudes about health for planning health services for them? An opportunity recently presented itself to examine some aspects of these questions in the Washington Heights section of New York City. . . . Youngsters were asked: "What do you see as some of the biggest health and medical problems for young people like yourself living around here?" This was a free answer question—no categories of response were suggested; rather, it was up to the youngster to decide what he considered to be a health or medical problem. Responses showed considerable agreement as to what the major adolescent health problems are: cigarette smoking (44%), drugs (34%), drinking (32%), and air pollution (18%).

From AJPH, *September 1969, pp. 1730–1734.*

How Three Clinical Professions Addressed Disability in Recent Decades

Daniel Fox, PhD, and James M. Perrin, MD

ABOUT THE AUTHORS

Daniel Fox is with the Milbank Memorial Fund, New York, NY. James M. Perrin is with MassGeneral Hospital for Children and Harvard Medical School, Boston, MA.

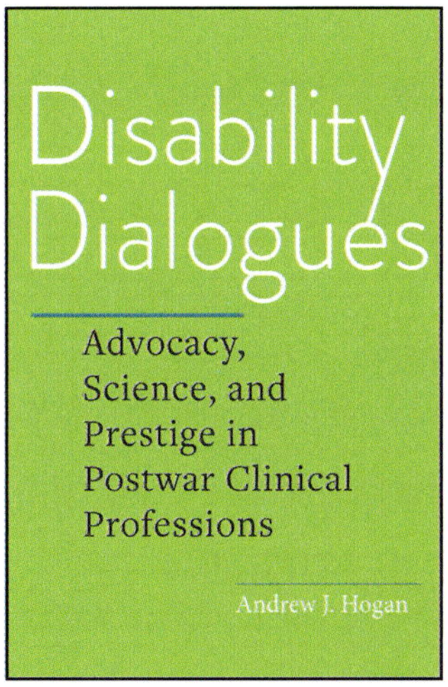

Disability Dialogues: Advocacy, Science, and Prestige in Postwar Clinical Professions
By Andrew J. Hogan
Baltimore, MD: Johns Hopkins University Press; 2022
Hardcover, xiii+246 pp.; $55.00
ISBN-13: 978-1421445335

Andrew Hogan's *Disability Dialogues* provides an interesting recent history of three related professions and changes in their experience of disability, evolving scientific approach and theory, inclusion of people with disabilities, and approach to environmental and political disability issues. The three professions—psychology, genetics (emphasizing genetic counselors), and pediatrics—share some joint interest in the assessment and care of people with disabilities but also vary a good deal in their places in the broader health and public health communities.

ORGANIZATION AND SCOPE OF THE BOOK

The book opens with a brief history of the high rates of institutionalization of people with disabilities until about the mid-1950s, followed by growing momentum and varied capacity for care in communities. Of interest, another professional group, psychiatry, played a major role in institutional care, generally leading the institution staff and defining most institutional policies. Hogan does not discuss sufficiently the continuing role of psychiatrists with people with disabilities after deinstitutionalization, suggesting that these other professions (as well as other groups in clinical medicine) replaced them. Partly, this reflects the author's view of disability as mainly physical and intellectual. Psychiatry has maintained substantial roles, especially with such conditions as autism and more serious behavioral disorders. Autism could have been an interesting inclusion because it brings in different interactions among the clinical disciplines and highlights other developmental aspects of the fields.

Hogan describes well the growing biomedical and other research advances in numerous conditions that are associated with disability. He notes how these advances also conflicted with inclusion of people with disabilities in all aspects of their care, a tension that he characterizes as between scientific rigor and the inclusion of people with disabilities in making decisions where the science might not provide guidance. He also notes intraprofessional conflicts between individual clinical approaches and sociopolitical strategies to improve the social environment and lessen stigmatization of people with disabilities.

Hogan makes good efforts to compare and contrast the three professions, although, in reality, they faced similar challenges and tensions as they worked toward greater inclusion of people with disabilities in many aspects of care and policy. He also documents well the controversies within the professions, and how key leaders moved toward change, often meeting much opposition or no interest among colleagues. It might help to delve a bit further into issues in the philosophy of science of the professions (especially psychiatry), where definitions of science and evidence differ and, of course, the scientific foci are quite different. Disciplinary definitions and their

AJPH August 2023, Vol 113, No. 8

evolution very much influence how the professions changed with new science in their portfolios, including evidence arising from the inclusion of people with disabilities in their own care. Debates over evidence much influenced official positions of professional organizations.

All three groups faced much internal discussion of the growing sociopolitical understanding of disability, in combination with efforts by people with disabilities to band together and demand change in aspects of their daily lives and environments as well as a greater role in their care—what interventions they received, assessment of results, and how decisions were made. All three professions moved over time to much greater inclusion for people with disabilities. Some changes came from people with disabilities within each profession, although much came from organized groups of people with disabilities or their parents and caregivers. Debates within the professions, including about the training of professionals, generally slowed progress. Genetic counselors have a somewhat different developmental history, given their early history as helping staff for clinical geneticists but then increasing development of standards and defined responsibilities of counselors, crafting new responsibilities and expanding services families received. Here, interesting debates evolved about the scope and responsibilities of counselors and their independence, as well as their roles in social and environmental changes.

LEADERSHIP

The book helpfully describes several key figures in all three groups who raised attention to the issues of disability, often as a result of personal experience with family members with disability. With the growing empowerment of people with disabilities in these professions, numerous people with disabilities became leading advocates and teachers within the professions and helped move attention to inclusion and sociopolitical support. The growing organized community of people with disabilities produced influential leaders. Hogan writes that these leaders, such as Adrienne Asch (and the late Judy Heumann), set their sights within one profession (here, genetic counseling), whereas many like Asch had impact on leaders in all three groups.

Hogan focuses the pediatric history mainly around a few key early leaders and then the difficult dispute between factions emphasizing neurodevelopmental disabilities and developmental and behavioral pediatrics. This helpful analysis describes tensions again between views of science as well as the scope of any definition of disability. Indeed, neither group has built a strong and effective network of support, leaving many children and their parents without satisfactory care. Whether more collaboration and compromise between these two factions would have led to a much stronger profession is a relevant speculation.

EXPANDING ROLE OF PEDIATRICS

During this period of dispute, nonetheless, pediatrics as a profession did expand its work in other ways, especially initially including parents of children with disabilities in their work and later younger people themselves. Increasing meaningful inclusion of parents in the work of pediatrics did take time but led to much change in the profession. An early policy study at Vanderbilt, led jointly by a psychologist and a pediatrician, highlighted common threads across diverse pediatric conditions and brought public health and policy attention to children with disabilities and their families. The leading pediatric organization, the American Academy of Pediatrics, produced numerous policy statements regarding inclusion and political advocacy for children and families, including expanding social roles and education. Fruitful interactions with parents began in the 1980s (some documented in the text) and expanded over time. Family Voices leaders had much involvement in moving this agenda. Asch and other advocates also had substantial influence on pediatric leadership (as well as psychology and genetics). And while internal professional battles took place in a segment of pediatrics, the book's discussion of Down syndrome notes that generalist and specialist pediatricians had much collaboration here with those in genetic counseling.

OTHER UNADDRESSED QUESTIONS

Other questions not addressed include these: How did these groups figure in the sociopolitical and public health advances related to disability? What role did they play in the development of the Americans with Disabilities Act and other key policy advances? How about various public support programs, such as Home and Community Based Services (or Medicaid more broadly) or the Supplemental Security Income program or Social Security Disability Insurance? For example, controversies over the past 25 to 30 years regarding the inclusion of children and youths with long-term mental health conditions has brought advocacy mainly from pediatrics and some from psychology. Psychiatry has been generally absent from these debates and related policy efforts.

A discussion of the relationship of public health theory and practice to the management of care for persons with disabilities would have been useful. The author mentions only a few public health professionals and one graduate program (and not until p. 58). Moreover, there are no citations to the literature on the relationship.[1] Similarly, Hogan does not discuss why the state agencies that housed and managed the outpatient care of most persons with disabilities were separate from state departments of health.

Overall, the book offers good perspectives of how the psychology, genetics (emphasizing genetic counselors), and pediatrics professions increasingly engaged people with disabilities in their professions and in decision-making about their care. AJPH

CORRESPONDENCE

Correspondence should be sent to Daniel M. Fox, 100 W 12th St, Apt 3T, New York, NY 10011-8242 (e-mail: dmfox@milbank.org). Reprints can be ordered at https://ajph.org by clicking the "Reprints" link.

PUBLICATION INFORMATION

Full Citation: Fox D, Perrin JM. How three clinical professions addressed disability in recent decades. *Am J Public Health*. 2023;113(8):829–831.
Acceptance Date: April 6, 2023.
DOI: https://doi.org/10.2105/AJPH.2023.307314

CONTRIBUTORS

The authors contributed equally to writing this review.

CONFLICTS OF INTEREST

The authors have no conflicts of interest to disclose.

REFERENCE

1. Wilber N, Mitra M, Walker DK, Allen D, Meyers AR, Tupper P. Disability as a public health issue: findings and reflections from the Massachusetts Survey of Secondary Conditions. *Milbank Q*. 2002;80(2): 393–421. https://doi.org/10.1111/1468-0009.00009

Winning Rights: The Role of Worker Centers in Protecting the Most Vulnerable Workers

Marcy Goldstein-Gelb, MS, and Luz S. Marin, ScD

ABOUT THE AUTHORS

Marcy Goldstein-Gelb is co-executive director of the National Council for Occupational Safety and Health (National COSH), Somerville, MA. Luz S. Marin is an associate professor in the Department of Safety Sciences, Indiana University of Pennsylvania, Indiana, PA.

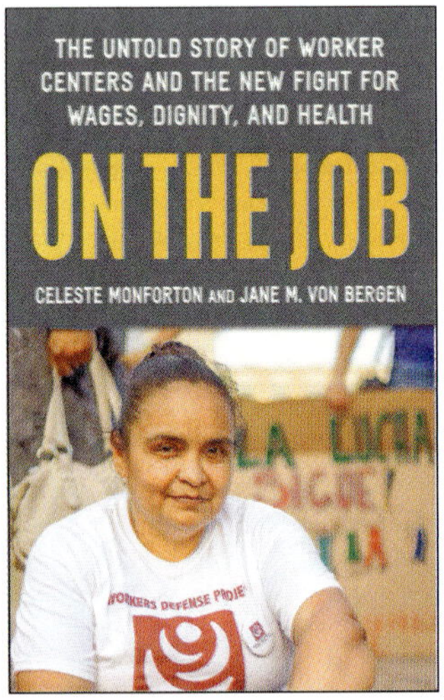

On the Job: The Untold Story of Worker Centers and the New Fight for Wages, Dignity, and Health
By Celeste Monforton and Jane M. Von Bergen
New York, NY: The New Press; 2021
Hardcover, 288 pp; $26.99
ISBN: 978-1-62097-501-5

For millions of workers in America, simply trying to earn a living means enduring dangerous working conditions, underpayment of wages, or harassment on a daily basis. Workers with the fewest job options—because of immigration status, education, and systemic racism—often are subjected to the harshest work conditions and have the most to lose if they speak up. Exercising workers' rights, including receiving fair compensation for the work done or having a safe and healthy working environment, is not the norm for a large portion of workers in the United States. Even worse, some workers, such as domestic workers, have been excluded from coverage by labor laws.[1] In great need of a safe space to address poor conditions, workers are increasingly turning to community-based organizations known as worker centers.[2–4]

Celeste Monforton and Jane M. Von Bergen's book, *On the Job: The Untold Story of Worker Centers and the New Fight for Wages, Dignity, and Health*, captures the story of workers fed up with toiling in dangerous jobs for paltry pay and of being forced to choose between their health and well-being or putting food on their table. It tells the story of a workforce not protected by a union collective bargaining agreement but able to assert its collective power through a growing part of the labor movement: worker centers. Worker centers began to emerge in the late 1970s and early 1980s, led by Black worker activists in North Carolina and South Carolina and immigrant activists in New York City and along the Texas–Mexico border. As of late 2021 they had grown to number over 246, funded by a combination of foundations, government, earned income, grassroots fundraising, and dues.[2]

Divided into seven insightful sections, the book discusses the role of worker centers as safe places for workers who have been exploited, abused and harassed, and robbed of their wages and dignity. They also describe the process of educating them about their rights and building power through collective action.

THE INTERSECTION OF WORKER SAFETY AND WORKER POWER

On the Job takes the reader across the country, describing the path of workers, mostly immigrants, who became workers' organizers after experiencing unfair conditions in their workplace. Workers like Mirella Nava, a Houston, Texas–based warehouse worker who became a worker center advocate after experiencing as a temporary worker exposure to dangerous chemicals and seeing firsthand how injured workers were not allowed to leave the workplace to receive medical attention until they "get the machine working again." Mirella and her coworkers gained support and community through the Fe y Justicia Worker Center, where they learned how to recognize hazards, make formal complaints to the Occupational Safety and Health Administration (OSHA), and guarantee that their voices would be heard in their own language by ensuring that a bilingual (English–Spanish) OSHA inspector led the claim investigation. As a member of the National Council for Occupational Safety and Health (National COSH), a network of 25 worker centers, the Fe y Justicia Worker Center in turn engages its worker members and organizers in a national community of learning, collaboration, and action.

WORKER CENTERS AND THEIR OWN CHALLENGES

Turning workers seeking help with a job problem into leaders and advocates is the key role of a worker center but also its major struggle. The book examines the tension created by the worker centers' constant endeavor to reach a balance between providing services to individuals and building workplace and community power. Resources and collaborations are key for keeping these centers working; fundraising, alliances, grant funding, and charging membership dues contribute to making the centers financially sustainable. The intense work that the centers do in different areas (e.g., immigration, wages, education, training, research, assessments) requires skillful leaders and organizers in many areas. Although motivated by their commitment to "being agents of social change," worker centers experienced high turnover among their leaders and organizers because of physical and emotional work demands. Despite their own struggles, the energy and commitment of people working in these centers has contributed to improved lives for thousands of workers. If not for *On the Job*, we might not be aware of their victories.

THE FRUITS OF THEIR LABORS

Worker centers also have a long track record of identifying patterns of workplace abuses and engaging their members in identifying and fighting for public policy solutions. Policy campaigns often start locally and then, by connecting with other local and state campaigns, become a national movement. *On the Job* highlights two examples of this local to national effort: the Domestic Worker Bill of Rights and the Temporary Worker Rights campaigns. Both campaigns sought to address widespread abuses affecting immigrants and people of color—women of color in particular, in the case of domestic workers. They were successful because they employed worker-centered approaches: engaging workers as leaders in conducting surveys to document conditions, sharing their stories and experiences, and issuing reports to bring workers' experiences out of the shadows and into the public discourse. *On the Job* highlights the importance of workers being both leaders for change and actively engaged in the enforcement of their implementation.

THE POWER AWAKENED

The COVID-19 pandemic revealed long-standing inadequate protections, inequities, and injustice for workers in US workplaces. Workers who have always been essential, providing us with goods and services that keep us alive, have long been canaries in the coal mine—toiling in dangerous conditions, with inadequate safety protections or without a financial safety net to tide them through an emergency. As *On the Job* recounts, during this crisis, workers turned to worker centers to build community leadership and demand urgently needed safety protections and paid time off. They engaged in collective action; for example, a car caravan, supported by the Greater Minnesota Worker Center, with chants of "Keep me safe at work" and "Essential not disposable." The strength and courage that workers demonstrated during COVID-19 sends a message that they will continue to demand their right to safety, to their hard-earned wages, and to justice—and that worker centers will continue to be there for them in sickness and in health. AJPH

CORRESPONDENCE

Correspondence should be sent to Luz S. Marin, ScD, 1010 Oakland Ave, Indiana, PA 15704 (e-mail: Luz.Marin@iup.edu). Reprints can be ordered at http://www.ajph.org by clicking the "Reprints" link.

PUBLICATION INFORMATION

Full Citation: Goldstein-Gelb M, Marin LS. Winning rights: the role of worker centers in protecting the most vulnerable workers. *Am J Public Health*. 2023;113(8):832–833.

Acceptance Date: May 17, 2023.

DOI: https://doi.org/10.2105/AJPH.2023.307345

CONTRIBUTORS

Both authors contributed equally to this review.

CONFLICTS OF INTEREST

The authors declare no competing financial interests.

REFERENCES

1. National Labor Relations Board. About NLRB. Are you covered? 2023. Available at: https://www.nlrb.gov/about-nlrb/rights-we-protect/the-law/employees/are-you-covered#:~:text=Excluded%20from%20coverage%20under%20the,the%20Railway%20Labor%20Act%2C%20and. Accessed April 2023.
2. Fine JR. *Worker Centers: Organizing Communities at the Edge of the Dream*. Ithaca, NY: Cornell University Press; 2006.
3. Theodore N, Valenzuela A, Meléndez E. Worker centers: defending labor standards for migrant workers in the informal economy. *Int J Manpow*. 2009;30(5):422–436. https://doi.org/10.1108/01437720910977634
4. Griffith KL. Worker centers and labor law protections: why aren't they having their cake? *Berkeley J Employ Labor Law*. 2015;36(331):331–349.

Improvements in Sexual Orientation and Gender Identity Data Collection Through Policy and Education

Marina Stasenko, MD, and Gwendolyn P. Quinn, PhD

ABOUT THE AUTHORS

Marina Stasenko and Gwendolyn P. Quinn are with the Department of Obstetrics and Gynecology and the Perlmutter Cancer Center at the Grossman School of Medicine, New York University, New York, NY.

See also Liu et al., p. 883.

AJPH August 2023, Vol 113, No. 8

Social determinants of health are nonmedical factors that can influence health outcomes and quality of life.[1] While extensive research has been conducted corroborating that race and economic stability profoundly affect one's health outcomes, there is still debate on other socioeconomic factors that may play a vital role, such as sexual orientation and gender identity (SOGI). The collection of social determinants of health data for medical care is slowly expanding and is shaped by public policy. In turn, public policy is shaped by data derived from the health care system. However, the dearth of data collection on SOGI, as well as other potentially pertinent patient demographics, limits their applicability and usability.

SEXUAL ORIENTATION AND GENDER IDENTITY DEMOGRAPHICS

Sexual and gender minority (SGM) status has been overlooked as fundamentally important to understanding a patient's health status. It was only in 2015 that the National Institutes of Health identified SGM persons as a population experiencing health disparities. SGM status includes "individuals who identify as lesbian, gay, bisexual, asexual, transgender, Two-Spirit, queer, and/or intersex" and accounts for approximately 10 million US adults.[2] SGM persons face unique challenges that lead to health disparities: higher rates of obesity and smoking, discrimination within the health care system, lower rates of private health insurance, and exclusion from traditional cancer screening campaigns.[3] Exact statistics on rates of diseases in SGM populations are difficult to ascertain, as SOGI data have traditionally not been collected by medical systems or large health care databases. For example, a survey of members of the American Society of Clinical Oncology noted that only approximately 40% of respondents collected SOGI data.[4] The National Cancer Institute's Surveillance, Epidemiology, and End Results database does not catalog SOGI data at all.

In an effort to improve clinical care for and clinical research about SGM patients, leading societies, including the National Institutes of Health and the Joint Commission, have emphasized the importance of collecting SOGI data as part of providing patient-centered care.[5–7] To address the lack of SOGI collection data by population-level databases, the Department of Health and Human Services Healthy People 2020 included SOGI data collection as an objective of the initiative.[8]

SEXUAL ORIENTATION AND GENDER IDENTITY AS REQUIRED DATA

In 2016, the US Health Resources and Services Administration decreed the collection of SOGI data by federally qualified health centers. Liu et al. (p. 883) examined the performance of SOGI data collection of the federally qualified health centers in their article in this issue. Their analyses showed that for sexual orientation, missing data decreased from 77.1% in 2016 to 29.1% in 2020–2021, and gender identity missing data fell from 68.2% to 24.0% over that period. Interestingly, data collection varied by state and racial demographics of the served patient population. Health centers in the South of the United States and those that care for more low-income or Black patient populations were more likely to have SOGI data collection.

The authors attribute this dramatic reduction in a six-year time span to introduction of SOGI data fields in the electronic medical record and the overarching mandate, creating a more favorable environment for data collection. Educating staff on the importance of SOGI data collection was also key to achieving the goal of decreasing missing data. This success was the culmination of the efforts and time investment of a multitude of organizations.

Patients reporting their SOGI demographics to clinicians results in more positive direct and indirect health outcomes and is associated with increased patient satisfaction and better self-reported health.[9] Furthermore, patients want to provide this information: one survey found that while 80% of providers felt that sexual orientation data collection would be offensive to their patients, only 11% of patients felt that they would be offended if questioned.[10]

As Liu et al. have shown, a clinical mandate combined with education and electronic tools to simplify collection can drastically improve rates of SOGI data collection. With that accomplished, the next step is to use those data to improve the health outcomes for this marginalized patient population. This will require training of health care clinicians in not only the collection of SOGI data but also the application of collected data to the care of the patients. While SOGI data collection is key to improving the health of SGM, it is not merely the collection of such data but rather skilled application of this information to provide patient-centered care. Best practices for training health care teams to apply SOGI data to patient care have been developed and include the need for focus on adult learning and evaluating the impact of training.[11] It is now time to put those practices into action to create a health care system that addresses the needs of our most vulnerable patients. AJPH

CORRESPONDENCE

Correspondence should be sent to Gwendolyn Quinn, 550 1st Ave, NBV 9N1-F, New York, NY 10016 (e-mail: gwendolyn.quinn@nyulangone.org). Reprints can be ordered at https://ajph.org by clicking the "Reprints" link.

PUBLICATION INFORMATION

Full Citation: Stasenko M, Quinn GP. Improvements in sexual orientation and gender identity data collection through policy and education. *Am J Public Health*. 2023;113(8):834–835.

Acceptance Date: May 16, 2023.

DOI: https://doi.org/10.2105/AJPH.2023.307344

CONTRIBUTORS

M. Stasenko and G. P. Quinn conceptualized, wrote, and edited this editorial.

CONFLICTS OF INTEREST

Both authors have no conflicts of interest.

REFERENCES

1. Brennan Ramirez LK, Baker EA, Metzler M. *Promoting Health Equity: A Resource to Help Communities Address Social Determinants of Health.* Atlanta, GA: US Department of Health and Human Services, Centers for Disease Control and Prevention; 2008.
2. Gates GJ. In US, more adults identifying as LGBT. 2017. Available at: http://www.gallup.com/poll/201731/lgbt-identification-rises.aspx?version=print. Accessed May 7, 2023.
3. Griggs J, Maingi S, Blinder V, et al. American Society of Clinical Oncology Position Statement: Strategies for reducing cancer health disparities among sexual and gender minority populations. *J Clin Oncol.* 2017;35(19):2203–2208. https://doi.org/10.1200/JCO.2016.72.0441
4. Kamen CS, Pratt-Chapman ML, Meersman SC, et al. Sexual orientation and gender identity data collection in oncology practice: findings of an ASCO survey. *JCO Oncol Pract.* 2022;18(8):e1297–e1305. https://doi.org/10.1200/OP.22.00084
5. Institute of Medicine. The health of lesbian, gay, bisexual, and transgender (LGBT) people: building a foundation for better understanding. Washington, DC: National Academies Press; 2011. https://doi.org/10.17226/13128
6. Deutsch MB, Green J, Keatley J, et al. Electronic medical records and the transgender patient: recommendations from the World Professional Association for Transgender Health EMR Working Group. *J Am Med Inform Assoc.* 2013;20(4):700–703. https://doi.org/10.1136/amiajnl-2012-001472
7. Deutsch MB, Buchholz D. Electronic health records and transgender patients—practical recommendations for the collection of gender identity data. *J Gen Intern Med.* 2015;30(6):843–847. https://doi.org/10.1007/s11606-014-3148-7
8. Office of Disease Prevention and Health Promotion. Lesbian, gay, bisexual, and transgender health. Healthy People 2020. Available at: https://wayback.archive-it.org/5774/20220413182850/https://www.healthypeople.gov/2020/topics-objectives/topic/lesbian-gay-bisexual-and-transgender-health. Accessed May 7, 2023.
9. Ruben MA, Fullerton M. Proportion of patients who disclose their sexual orientation to health-care providers and its relationship to patient outcomes: a meta-analysis and review. *Patient Educ Couns.* 2018;101(9):1549–1560. https://doi.org/10.1016/j.pec.2018.05.001
10. Maragh-Bass AC, Torain M, Adler R, et al. Risks, benefits, and importance of collecting sexual orientation and gender identity data in healthcare settings: a multi-method analysis of patient and provider perspectives. *LGBT Health.* 2017;4(2):141–152. https://doi.org/10.1089/lgbt.2016.0107
11. Pratt-Chapman ML, Eckstrand K, Robinson A, et al. Developing standards for cultural competency training for health care providers to care for lesbian, gay, bisexual, transgender, queer, intersex, and asexual persons: consensus recommendations from a national panel. *LGBT Health.* 2022;9(5):340–347. https://doi.org/10.1089/lgbt.2021.0464

Vaccinating the Masses During a Pandemic: Learning in Real Time for Tomorrow

Heather M. Brandt, PhD

ABOUT THE AUTHOR

Heather M. Brandt is the director of the HPV Cancer Prevention Program and full member in the Department of Epidemiology and Cancer Control at St. Jude Children's Research Hospital, Memphis, TN.

See also McColloch et al., p. 909.

AJPH August 2023, Vol 113, No. 8

Since March 2020, the COVID-19 pandemic has challenged the established public health infrastructure and systems in the United States and spurred innovation to meet the demands of the pandemic. The pandemic traversed phases of building awareness, securing personal protective equipment, ramping up of testing and surveillance, and launching treatment. The vaccination phase was rolled out beginning in late 2020 in the United States. We witnessed remarkable and exciting developments in efforts to slow and stop the pandemic in the form of COVID-19 vaccines. Many years of previous research, including past developments in mRNA vaccines and knowing how to sequence severe acute respiratory syndrome coronavirus 2 (SARS-CoV-2), led to the ability to develop and test vaccines for safety and effectiveness quickly in response. Distribution of COVID-19 vaccines was unprecedented on a global scale and posed implementation challenges that exceeded public health preparedness and planning.[1] There were several aspects of COVID-19 vaccination programs that should promote stronger preparation for the future.

McColloch et al. (p. 909) examined implementation of COVID-19 vaccinations at high-throughput—or mass—vaccination sites to understand how these sites implemented federal guidance and captured promising practices to inform similar sites now and in the future. The authors evaluated 134 high-throughput COVID-19 vaccination sites and community vaccination clinics across 30 immunization programs in the United States. The resulting promising practices centered on six themes:

1. addressing health equity,
2. leveraging partnerships,
3. optimizing site design and flow,
4. communicating through visual cues,
5. using quick response codes, and
6. prioritizing risk management and quality control.

These promising practices offer insight into the ways in which our implementation planning and execution can be improved in the future. However, we need more publications, reports, and sharing of lessons learned to be better prepared in the future. We also need to consider the role of vaccines, equity, and available, rigorous methods to ensure we are better prepared.

UNLIKE PREVIOUS VACCINES

Effective and efficient vaccine implementation is contingent on supply, delivery, storage, and administration in consideration of the context and conditions of implementation. It was clear that we would be unable to rely on the usual health care delivery system for COVID-19 vaccines in the United States.[2] The first two available COVID-19 vaccines were not the same as seasonal influenza, smallpox vaccine, or polio vaccines of past mass vaccination campaigns. As one example, the storage requirements of the two mRNA vaccines initially limited the settings in which people could access vaccines and posed implementation challenges. However, these challenges were addressed through coordinated planning between the US Centers for Disease Control and Prevention (CDC), Federal Emergency Management Agency, and state and local public health departments and immunization programs. In addition, the administration requirements of COVID-19 vaccinations during this first phase of rollout fostered novel partnerships, such as with a fast-food chain manager in South Carolina[3] who was called in to assist with logistics of a mass vaccination site, and applications of Lean principles and tools in Florida to improve efficiency and productivity and accelerate vaccination coverage[4] through mass vaccination efforts. The circumstances demanded a level of creativity unlike previous vaccination campaigns.

ENSURING VACCINATION FOR ALL

Vaccines in cold storage or a refrigerator do little good if people are unvaccinated. "Vaccines don't save lives; vaccinations save lives"[5] is a simple, yet powerful, way to convey merely having a vaccine—or in this case vaccines—available does not equal receipt. The so-called "last mile" of vaccine development is actual delivery in the form of vaccinations. According to the most recent COVID-19 vaccinations in the US data from the CDC,[6] 81.4% of people have been vaccinated with at least one dose, 69.5% have completed the primary series, and 17.0% have had the updated (bivalent) booster dose. There is great variation by geographic region and among certain population groups. What has overwhelmingly been highlighted in each phase of the pandemic and since initial introduction of the vaccines is the inequitable burden members of groups and populations that have been minoritized, marginalized, and underserved have faced in terms of disease burden (including death), lack of access to risk mitigation, and now vaccination.[7] If we want to understand these observed differences in vaccination coverage, we must invest in understanding factors influencing vaccination and plan accordingly with our efforts.[8] Equity must be fundamental to every action we undertake to ensure vaccination for all.

APPLYING IMPLEMENTATION SCIENCE TO THE LAST MILE

The National Cancer Institute definition of implementation science is "the study of methods to promote the adoption and integration of evidence-based practices, interventions, and policies into routine health care and public health settings to improve the impact on population health."[9] COVID-19 vaccination, an evidence-based intervention, offered us a highly effective approach to prevent serious disease, hospitalizations, and deaths. We know what to do and what health outcomes we can influence. However, going from "what" to outcomes is not linear and is not a path free of barriers.

We know myriad factors across multiple levels influence how we get from "what" to health outcomes. We may know "what" we want to implement, and we may know the outcome we want to achieve. It is what lies between "what" and health outcomes that is less well understood and studied—and it is the "how" part of the process or the strategies we use to get what we know works into widespread practice. The "how" is the piece that speaks to implementation strategies,[10] and the synergistic influences of inner and outer settings in which the "what" may be implemented. This is where implementation science comes into play. In this case, capacity, disinformation, vaccination hesitancy, and implementation processes and outcomes, such as supply of vaccines, funding and other resources, equity and inclusion, messaging and communication, and access points factored in to how we were able to deliver on the last mile.

The COVID-19 pandemic significantly stressed public health systems around the world and exposed gaps in health care for underserved and vulnerable populations. Public health system preparedness is paramount for protecting the health of all. This will require intentionality and advanced planning, including engaging those who have not historically been a part of the process and employing ingenuity. Mass vaccination approaches were highly acceptable[11] and have largely disappeared two years after introduction in the United States. Implementation science offers us a rigorous way to understand and accommodate key determinants in our implementation strategies to yield optimal levels of vaccination for all. We must invest resources to ensure we have the public health capacity to convert vaccines to vaccinations rapidly in the future. We can do this by acting now to improve access to vaccinations during the booster phase (and first dose for some) by meeting people where they are, helping people make informed decisions, and building confidence and trust in vaccinations through effective and trusted messaging. It is a matter of when, not if, we will face the next pandemic. It is up to us—as a global public health community—to facilitate and support information sharing and engage in courageous conversations about what worked well and what did not and who was left behind in the process. AJPH

CORRESPONDENCE

Correspondence should be sent to Heather M. Brandt, PhD, Director, HPV Cancer Prevention Program, St. Jude Children's Research Hospital, 262 Danny Thomas Place, Memphis, TN 38105 (e-mail: heather.brandt@stjude.org). Reprints can be ordered at http://ajph.org by clicking the "Reprints" link.

PUBLICATION INFORMATION

Full Citation: Brandt HM. Vaccinating the masses during a pandemic: learning in real time for tomorrow. *Am J Public Health*. 2023;113(8):836–838.
Acceptance Date: May 23, 2023.
DOI: https://doi.org/10.2105/AJPH.2023.307358

ACKNOWLEDGMENTS

This publication was supported by the American Lebanese and Syrian Associated Charities (ALSAC) of St. Jude Children's Research Hospital.

CONFLICTS OF INTEREST

The author reports no conflicts of interest.

REFERENCES

1. Wilensky GR. 2020 revealed how poorly the US was prepared for COVID-19 and future pandemics. *JAMA*. 2021;325(11):1029–1030. https://doi.org/10.1001/jama.2021.1046
2. Goralnick E, Kaufmann C, Gawande AA. Mass-vaccination sites—an essential innovation to curb the COVID-19 pandemic. *N Engl J Med*. 2021;384(18):e67. https://doi.org/10.1056/NEJMp2102535

3. Fowler H. Chick-Fil-A manager lends drive-thru skills to COVID vaccine site in South Carolina. *The State*. January 27, 2021. Available at: https://www.thestate.com/news/state/south-carolina/article248803035.html. Accessed May 21, 2023.
4. Froman MN, Walser MP, Lauzardo M, Graban M, Southwick FS. Applying Lean principles to create a high throughput mass COVID-19 vaccination site. *BMJ Open Qual.* 2022;11(1):e001617. https://doi.org/10.1136/bmjoq-2021-001617
5. Orenstein W. Vaccines don't save lives. Vaccinations save lives. *Hum Vaccin Immunother.* 2019;15(12):2786–2789. https://doi.org/10.1080/21645515.2019.1682360
6. Centers for Disease Control and Prevention. COVID data tracker. US Department of Health and Human Services. Available at: https://covid.cdc.gov/covid-data-tracker. Accessed May 21, 2023.
7. Labgold K, Hamid S, Shah S, et al. Estimating the unknown: greater racial and ethnic disparities in COVID-19 burden after accounting for missing race and ethnicity data. *Epidemiology.* 2021;32(2):157–161. https://doi.org/10.1097/EDE.0000000000001314
8. Cunningham-Erves J, George W, Stewart EC, et al. COVID-19 vaccination: comparison of attitudes, decision-making processes, and communication among vaccinated and unvaccinated Black Americans. *Int J Environ Res Public Health.* 2023;20(4):3481. https://doi.org/10.3390/ijerph20043481
9. National Cancer Institute. About implementation science. Available at: https://cancercontrol.cancer.gov/is/about#:~:text=Implementation%20science%20(IS)%20is%20the,our%20impact%20on%20population%20health. Accessed May 21, 2023.
10. Proctor EK, Landsverk J, Aarons G, Chambers D, Glisson C, Mittman B. Implementation research in mental health services: an emerging science with conceptual, methodological, and training challenges. *Adm Policy Ment Health.* 2009;36(1):24–34. https://doi.org/10.1007/s10488-008-0197-4
11. Danek S, Büttner M, Krois J, Schwendicke F. How do users respond to mass vaccination centers? A cross-sectional study using natural language processing on online reviews to explore user experience and satisfaction with COVID-19 vaccination centers. *Vaccines (Basel).* 2023;11(1):144. https://doi.org/10.3390/vaccines11010144

Data Democratization for Health Equity: A Public Health of Consequence, August 2023

Farzana Kapadia, PhD, MPH

ABOUT THE AUTHOR

Farzana Kapadia is the deputy editor of AJPH and is an associate professor of epidemiology at the School of Global Public Health, New York University, New York.

See also Jamal et al., p. 852, and Liu et al., p. 883.

The increasing speed of availability, volume, and complexity of data accessible to public health professionals are paralleled by rapid developments in software programs and applications with cutting-edge computational abilities to manage data. Ideally, the product of these advancements will have powerful potential for affecting population health. For example, from a surveillance perspective, using multisectoral data would provide timely information on population health status and improve our knowledge and understanding of how health inequities are shaped by social, economic, and political forces.[1]

From public health and health policy perspectives, these data would guide where, when, and how to apply policies and practices that would narrow health inequities. It is clear that early in the COVID-19 pandemic the lack of timely, accurate, and accessible data limited public health's ability to determine what local action would avert substantial COVID-19–related morbidity and mortality. As the COVID-19 pandemic evolved, the proliferating data dashboards—at federal, state, and local levels—for providing various types and layers of data on the physical, economic, social, and environmental conditions as drivers of COVID-19 became a mainstay.

Data dashboards are no longer confined to COVID-19: one can find them on opioid overdose[2] and HIV (https://ahead.hiv.gov), as just two examples. Yet, across these domains, challenges associated with developing, managing, and maintaining data dashboards persist and may undermine efforts that can ensure the true democratization of data.

DATA DEMOCRATIZATION

Understanding which agencies manage data collection systems, how they determine what data are collected, and whether, how, and to whom they make data accessible all play salient and significant roles in how data are used. At the same time, the people—and this means everyone—that we collect data from need to have clear assurances that their information will be used to improve their health and well-being, that it will be protected, and that it will be used with their interests at the forefront. In this issue of *AJPH*, we consider some of these key concerns with an eye to how the democratization of public health data can become a community asset in our march toward health justice and health equity.

DATA COLLECTION PRACTICES FOR EQUITY

Collection of data from minoritized and marginalized people involves ascertaining meaningful information with the goal of positively transforming the type and quality of clinical health care services, health promotion and prevention services, and socioeconomic resources that people want, need, and should receive. Increasingly, efforts are being made to collect information on the social determinants of health in clinical settings as well as in federal, state, and local data systems. These efforts, particularly with regard to collecting sexual orientation and gender identity (SOGI) data, highlight how thoughtful and careful data collection practices are necessary to enable sensitive but necessary data collection.

Following a Health Resources and Services Administration mandate that all federally qualified health centers collect SOGI data,[3] a 2016 review of SOGI collection at these centers revealed that 77.1%[4] of health center clients had no SOGI information in their electronic health records. Fast-forward, and in this issue of *AJPH*, Liu et al. (p. 883) report that sexual orientation was not collected on 29.1% of patients and gender identity on 24.0%. Importantly, as Liu et al. note, federally qualified health centers located in the Southern United States, which are more likely to be the usual source of health care for low-income and Black patients, were more likely to do better at collecting complete SOGI data. The authors attribute these gains in SOGI data collection—across all jurisdictions—to provider and clinical staff training efforts. This success does not rest on getting buy-in from clinical staff alone.

The foundation for these successes is honoring the specific and diverse communities served by federally qualified health centers and heeding their feedback on how to reduce provider and staff stigma and discrimination, ensure privacy of information, respect local norms, and translate SOGI data into information and practice that translates into health equity and health justice for LGBTQ+ (lesbian, gay, bisexual, transgender, and queer or questioning) patients. Moving forward, these practices will need to be flexible and consider how to incorporate and honor the diverse cultural backgrounds, languages, and evolving SOGI terminology that are specific to a given region or group. This will require striking a balance between uniformity of methodology and responsiveness to local communities.

DATA ACCESS FOR DATA EQUITY

As with efforts to enhance methods for collecting SOGI data, efforts to collect disaggregated data on Asian Americans, Native Hawaiians, and Pacific Islanders (AANHPIs) have gained momentum over the past decade. The challenges to the logistics of sampling and oversampling across disaggregated AANHPI groups persists, but a more pressing concern is the barrier to accessing these data. Although federal laws and policies governing the privacy and security of public health data are meant to protect the confidentiality of survey participants, these same policies can be significant barriers to gaining access to these data to identify and understand health inequities.

In this issue, Jamal et al. (p. 852) present an overview of federal disaggregated AANHPI data sets; yet, because of concerns regarding security and confidentiality, full and easy access to these data is restricted. Although protecting data is necessary, a lack of accessibility to disaggregated data undermines the ability to understand health inequities in and across AANHPI groups—groups that include vastly diverse linguistic, cultural, religious, and economic domains. The data use restrictions enumerated by Jamal et al. are not negligible and often involve significant costs and other logistical burdens that can prevent use. Once again, the call for striking a balance between protecting confidentiality and enabling data use is warranted. One way to manage data that may provide a pathway for greater data sharing is using the FAIR (Findable, Accessible, Interoperable, Reusable) guiding principles (https://www.go-fair.org/fair-principles). Indeed, such a framework could prove useful to achieving data equity and could become a pathway toward achieving health equity.

CONCLUSIONS

As we continue to compile meaningful data for public-facing dashboards, these dashboards' ability to be in tune with and meet the needs of communities and stakeholders relies on accurate and complete data collection of key social determinants of health and unrestricted access to the underlying data for the communities that they seek to profile.

Let us bear in mind that our goal is not to collect data for the sake of collecting data. Rather, we collect data to transform it into information, which grants us better knowledge and knowledge that provides guidance for evidence-based public health practices. Moreover, to achieve data equity, we need to be engaged with the communities from which these data arise to make sense of the data by understanding the context and human landscape they represent.

A public health of consequence rests on data equity, which encompasses the continuum from data collection to data access—if we are committed to seeing where health inequalities and injustices are present to end them. AJPH

CORRESPONDENCE

Correspondence should be sent to Farzana Kapadia, PhD, MPH, New York University, School of Global Public Health, 708 Broadway, Room 729, New York, NY 10003 (e-mail: farzana.kapadia@nyu.edu). Reprints can be ordered at http://www.ajph.org by clicking the "Reprints" link.

PUBLICATION INFORMATION

Full Citation: Kapadia F. Data democratization for health equity: a public health of consequence, August 2023. *Am J Public Health*. 2023;113(8):839–840.

Acceptance Date: May 21, 2023.

DOI: https://doi.org/10.2105/AJPH.2023.307350

CONFLICTS OF INTEREST

The author has no conflicts of interest to disclose.

REFERENCES

1. Thorpe LE, Chunara R, Roberts T, et al. Building Public Health Surveillance 3.0: emerging timely measures of physical, economic, and social environmental conditions affecting health. *Am J Public Health*. 2022;112(10):1436–1445. https://doi.org/10.2105/AJPH.2022.306917
2. Centers for Disease Control and Prevention. Drug overdose surveillance and epidemiology (DOSE) system. May 15, 2023. Available at: https://www.cdc.gov/drugoverdose/nonfatal/dashboard. Accessed May 23, 2023.
3. Streed CG Jr, Grasso C, Reisner SL, Mayer KH. Sexual orientation and gender identity data collection: clinical and public health importance. *Am J Public Health*. 2020;110(7):991–993. https://doi.org/10.2105/AJPH.2020.305722
4. Grasso C, Goldhammer H, Funk D, et al. Required sexual orientation and gender identity reporting by US health centers: first-year data. *Am J Public Health*. 2019;109(8):1111–1118. https://doi.org/10.2105/AJPH.2019.305130

East Palestine, Ohio, Railroad Derailment—Lessons to Learn, Actions to Take

C. Mary Schooling, PhD, Heidi E. Jones, PhD, and Suzanne McDermott, PhD

ABOUT THE AUTHORS

All authors are with the School of Public Health, City University of New York, New York.

East Palestine, Ohio, is the latest example of the creation of a preventable long-term health hazard for people and the planet.

On the evening of Friday, February 3, 2023, a Norfolk Southern Railroad freight train hauling 150 cars partly derailed in East Palestine because of wheel-bearing overheating. Some of the derailed cars spilled hazardous materials and sparked a fire that burned for days. On February 6, local residents were evacuated before Norfolk Southern Railroad undertook a controlled burn-off because of concerns that five of the derailed cars, which contained vinyl chloride, might explode. Vinyl chloride was released into a trough and set alight, generating a large pewter-colored plume of smoke that included phosgene and hydrogen chloride.

Currently, we do not know exactly what other chemical mixtures were released, although dioxin has been found. However, we do know that vinyl chloride is associated with an increased risk of hepatic angiosarcoma, hepatocellular carcinoma, brain and lung cancers, lymphoma, and leukemia. Phosgene was used as a chemical weapon in World War I to destroy soldiers' lungs, and dioxins are classified as a group 1 carcinogen that can affect male fertility. Dioxin can induce cancer years later, particularly in those exposed as babies or children and those heavily exposed, such as first responders.

It is imperative to rapidly evaluate exposures and establish a registry of people near the derailment. In addition to establishing full corporate accountability for the long-term health consequences to the surrounding community, we need to ensure that regulatory processes prevent any recurrence.

The train derailment at East Palestine was not inevitable; approximately 1000 derailments were reported in the United States during 2022 alone.[1] Train accidents are more common in the United States than in comparable countries despite fewer passenger miles and less freight transported.[2] The risk for train derailment and its consequences should have been avoided by better supervision and regulation by the Department of Transportation and the Environmental Protection Agency (EPA), respectively. The key issue is in whose interests these governmental bodies are acting. It is easy to assume that their only concern is to keep the public safe.

The United States has strong inequities in power, with wealthy individuals and corporations advocating deregulation in their own interests. Government agencies can be portrayed as overbearing and ineffective purveyors of "red tape" that stifles innovation, which adds fuel to a bonfire of regulations potentially leaving the rest of us at risk. Norfolk Southern Railroad was lobbying against "regulatory burdens," while advertising that "safety is a way of life and one of our guiding principles."[3] For example, a rule concerning advanced train braking technology was recently removed. Although this regulation may not have prevented the disaster in East Palestine, this type of deregulation indicates the direction of travel regulations. The US train industry has become increasingly less regulated over the past 40 years.[4]

The problem of how to regulate the regulators has been recognized since governments began using regulations to control behavior and was first articulated by the Roman poet Juvenal two millennia ago: "Who watches the watchers?"[5] Regulatory capture can undermine regulators if they act in the interests of the regulated industry rather than the public. Almost inevitably, vested interests win out over the public good, because they have more resources to influence regulators than the public. Alliances between industry representatives and regulators form over time, as personal relationships develop and opportunities arise to engage in conversations that modify the regulators' ability to enforce standards and question practices.

Often, when industries want to change the focus from harms to benefits to the public, they offer community services and incentives, such as creating parks and other recreational attractions. Northern Suffolk Railroad has proposed improvements to East Palestine Park.[6] This activity can distract the

AJPH August 2023, Vol 113, No. 8

public from the harms of industry practices.

By contrast, it is time consuming and difficult for advocacy organizations and scientists to obtain information and track events on an ongoing basis to ensure that regulations are developed and enforced and that data are collected to evaluate health consequences. However, a well-funded, well-staffed, transparent, independent regulator operating with clear principles, including a remit to serve the public, could do so and should be less open to regulatory capture[7]; however, such a regulator could be undermined by political appointments and processes.

Recently, regulatory capture at the EPA was documented and was predicted to reduce the EPA's ability "to confront polluting industries and promote public and environmental health."[8] It was also expected to have health consequences that "will likely fall hardest on vulnerable social groups, such as low-income communities, farmworkers and first responders,"[8(pS93)] as seen in East Palestine.

Taken together, regulatory capture and vested interests generate a "doom loop." Regulatory capture results in public agencies acting against the public interest and in the interests of capital gain by heads of industry, which promotes distrust and lack of support for the very institutions, such as the EPA, that are intended to promote the public interest. Vested interests siphon wealth to the rich, leaving less money for regulatory control and more risk to be suffered by everyone else, and hence more regulatory failure.

More monitoring of wheel bearings, removal of loose wheels, better braking technologies, more safety inspections, more staff, and less precision-scheduled railroading, and hence shorter trains, have all been suggested as ways of making the railroads safer. East Palestine was unlucky enough to be where a preventable environmental disaster occurred as a result of the current deregulated system. This event should serve as a wake-up call for us to act together to demand regulatory independence that acts in the public interest—the lives of our loved ones and the planet are at stake.

In this context of regulatory capture, the decision to have the controlled burn-off in East Palestine needs to be reviewed and the EPA appointment of Norfolk Southern Railroad to lead the cleanup rescinded. It is completely inappropriate for Norfolk Southern Railroad to be involved in the cleanup, as they obviously have a vested interest in minimizing the reporting of hazards, as illustrated by concerns about one of their contractors.[9] The EPA has appointed the fox to mind the hen house.

An independent body needs to be established that has a much wider remit than the EPA's cleanup. First, the exposures need to be characterized, the plume reconstructed, and the exposed populations of East Palestine, and elsewhere, enumerated for registry construction. Epidemiologists and community health professionals have the skills to establish such a registry and to conduct long-term monitoring, building on the Assessment of Chemical Exposure survey.[10]

Second, those affected need to be provided with monitoring to characterize health outcomes over time, as was done after 9/11 in New York City. Third, carcinogen exposures take time to result in detectable cancers, so East Palestine residents need guaranteed medical care into the future. All these activities must be implemented independent of but at the expense of Norfolk Southern Railroad. In this context, the refusal of Norfolk Southern Railroad to commit to long-term support for East Palestine is completely unacceptable.

Finally, we need to go back to the root causes of this accident in East Palestine and address them as well. First, we must reduce our reliance on hazardous chemicals and minimize their transport. Second, we need to treat the railways as a common good, like roads, which are run safely for the benefit of everyone. Third, we need watchdogs to identify, report, and combat regulatory capture. Fourth, we, as public health professionals, need to fight against regulatory capture and vested interests, do everything we can to address the situation in East Palestine, and ensure that such environmental disasters never recur. Taken together these actions should obviate the doom loop of regulatory capture and vested interests and create a healthier society and environment in the United States for everyone. AJPH

CORRESPONDENCE

Correspondence should be sent to Heidi E. Jones, 55 W 125th St, New York, NY 10027 (e-mail: heidi.jones@sph.cuny.edu). Reprints can be ordered at http://www.ajph.org by clicking the "Reprints" link.

PUBLICATION INFORMATION

Full Citation: Schooling CM, Jones HE, McDermott S. East Palestine, Ohio, railroad derailment—lessons to learn, actions to take. *Am J Public Health*. 2023;113(8):841–843.

Acceptance Date: May 20, 2023.

DOI: https://doi.org/10.2105/AJPH.2023.307353

CONTRIBUTORS

C. M. Schooling collated information and wrote the first draft of the editorial. H. E. Jones and S. McDermott conceptualized the editorial and reviewed it critically for important intellectual content. All authors approved the final version.

CONFLICTS OF INTEREST

The authors have no funding or affiliated interests and no other conflicts of interest to declare.

REFERENCES

1. Hernandez J. There are about 3 US train derailments per day. They aren't usually major disasters. March 9, 2023. Available at: https://www.npr.org/2023/03/09/1161921856/there-are-about-3-u-s-train-derailments-per-day-they-arent-usually-major-disaste. Accessed June 1, 2023.
2. Argon Data Visualization; Wikipedia. Countries with most number of rail accidents 2010–2019. Available at: https://www.getargon.io/posts/transportation/rail/top-countries-number-accidents-2010-2019. Accessed March 23, 2023.
3. Shaw A. CEO perspective: safety first, safety always. March 23, 2023. Available at: http://www.nscorp.com/content/nscorp/en/about-ns/safety.html. Accessed June 1, 2023.
4. Pierre-Louis K. How decades of lax rules enable train disasters. *Atlantic*. March 23, 2023. Available at: https://www.theatlantic.com/science/archive/2023/03/how-deregulation-enabled-train-disasters-like-east-palestine/673502. Accessed June 1, 2023.
5. Saltelli A, Dankel DJ, Di Fiore M, Holland N, Pigeon M. Science, the endless frontier of regulatory capture. *Futures*. 2022;135:102860. https://doi.org/10.1016/j.futures.2021.102860
6. Boney S. Norfolk Southern CEO back in East Palestine to discuss park improvements. March 30, 2023. Available at: https://www.newsbreak.com/east-palestine-oh/2975063281883-norfolk-southern-ceo-back-in-east-palestine-to-discuss-park-improvements. Accessed June 1, 2023.
7. Hempling S. "Regulatory capture": sources and solutions. *Governance and Accountability Review* 2014;1(1). Available at: https://scholarlycommons.law.emory.edu/cgi/viewcontent.cgi?article=1003&context=ecgar. Accessed June 1, 2023.
8. Dillon L, Sellers C, Underhill V, et al. The Environmental Protection Agency in the early Trump administration: prelude to regulatory capture. *Am J Public Health*. 2018;108(suppl 2):S89–S94. https://doi.org/10.2105/AJPH.2018.304360
9. Dayen D. The checkered past of the contractor monitoring the air in East Palestine. *American Prospect*. March 3, 2023. Available at: https://prospect.org/environment/2023-03-03-cteh-contractor-air-monitoring-east-palestine. Accessed June 1, 2023.
10. Centers for Disease Control and Prevention. CDC and ATSDR staff begin next steps in ACE investigation in East Palestine, Ohio. Available at: https://www.cdc.gov/media/releases/2023/p0313-chemical-exposure.html. Accessed June 1, 2023.

Where Was Climate Change at the White House Conference on Hunger, Nutrition, and Health?

Rachel G. Clark, JD, Sydney Pryor, MPH, and William H. Dietz, MD, PhD

ABOUT THE AUTHORS

The authors are with the Sumner M. Redstone Global Center for Prevention and Wellness, Milken Institute School of Public Health, George Washington University, Washington, DC.

In the fall of 2022, the Biden administration brought renewed attention to food insecurity and diet-related chronic disease by holding the first White House Conference on Hunger, Nutrition, and Health in more than 50 years. The administration has also made climate change a key focus by rejoining the Paris Climate Agreement, investing in climate adaptation and resilience, and committing to cutting greenhouse gas (GHG) emissions 50% to 52% below 2005 levels by 2030.[1] These actions appropriately prioritize the pressing public health threats posed by hunger, undernutrition, and climate change, but so far the administration has failed to recognize that these threats are closely interconnected. We cannot effectively nourish the population and prevent the irreversible environmental damages of climate change without making our food system more sustainable.[2,3] To succeed in meeting these twin objectives, the administration must align its food and nutrition priorities with its climate priorities.

IMPORTANCE OF A NATIONAL STRATEGY FOR FOOD AND CLIMATE

The White House Conference on Hunger, Nutrition, and Health, held on September 28, 2022, included the release of the Biden administration's National Strategy on Hunger, Nutrition, and Health, a "whole of government" approach to achieving the administration's stated objective of "ending hunger and increasing healthy eating and physical activity by 2030, so that fewer Americans experience diet-related chronic diseases like diabetes, obesity, and hypertension."[4] The national strategy comprises more than 140 actions organized into five pillars: improving food access and affordability, integrating nutrition and health, empowering all consumers to make and have access to healthy choices, supporting physical activity for all, and enhancing nutrition and food security research. Despite the existential threat of climate change to human and planetary health, there is only one reference to climate change and the food system in the entire report, and that reference focuses on the need for research rather than actionable strategies and policies that can be implemented today.

The link between climate change and the food system is undeniable.[5–7] By some estimates, food system activities, including food production, distribution, and disposal, produce a third of global GHG emissions caused by humans.[8] As a driver of climate change, the food system contributes to numerous public health threats, including severe weather events,[9] heat-related illness and death,[10] pollution and poor air quality,[11] vector-borne diseases,[12] and water-related illness.[13] At the same time, climate change threatens our ability to provide safe, good-quality food to all. The food system is vulnerable to the short- and long-term effects of climate change, such as severe weather events that cause disruptions to food supply chains.[14] Such disruptions also threaten access to safe drinking water, contributing to water insecurity, which is closely associated with food insecurity.[15]

Climate change contributes to undernutrition and diet-related diseases as well.[5] For instance, increased GHG emissions reduce crop yields and the micronutrient content of crops, both of which contribute to food and nutrition insecurity and undernutrition.[7] The disparate effects of diet-related chronic disease, food and nutrition insecurity, and adverse climate events suggest an immediate urgency to promote both sustainable and equitable food and nutrition policies.[16,17]

Despite these myriad connections, the Biden administration's national strategy does not recognize that climate change interacts with its goals

AJPH August 2023, Vol 113, No. 8

across all five pillars. Instead, the lone reference to climate change appears at the very end of the report, in the section on food security research. Stating that "climate change has direct relevance for the future of food security and human health," the administration commits to researching the effects of climate on food and nutrition security in two specific ways: the National Institutes of Health Climate and Health Initiative will assess the effects of climate change on food quality and nutrition security on the health of populations, and the US Department of Agriculture (USDA) will work with the National Academies of Sciences, Engineering, and Medicine to determine the links between human health and soil health.[4]

Although we are relieved to see at least one mention of the connection between food, climate, and health, research alone will not produce the transformative changes necessary to prevent and mitigate the urgent threats of climate change. Transformative changes require action driven by effective policies. The need for these policies was notably absent from the national strategy. The strategy also fails to acknowledge that the relationship between food and climate is bidirectional: not only does climate change threaten the quantity and quality of the food and water supply, but food production, processing, transport, consumption, and disposal also have a significant impact on climate and environmental degradation. There are immediate actions that the administration can take to align food policies and programs across agencies with its stated climate goals and to address the bidirectional threat of climate change and the food system, such as adding sustainability considerations to many of the actions already included in the national strategy.

INCREASE ACCESS TO HEALTHY AND SUSTAINABLE FOODS

Noting the prevalence of diet-related chronic diseases such as diabetes and heart disease, the national strategy includes several actions intended to improve the healthfulness of the American diet by increasing access to healthy food. But the report forgoes the opportunity to ensure that these policies encourage shifts toward both healthier and more sustainable options with lower GHG emissions. Agriculture, particularly the production of ruminant meats such as beef, is a major contributor to global GHG emissions; research suggests that we will not meet the goals of the Paris Climate Agreement without shifting our diets toward lower emission foods.[2,18,19] For this reason, the administration's strategies for healthy food access should incorporate climate considerations. Such policies would be mutually reinforcing because strong evidence indicates that a more sustainable diet is a healthier one.[2]

The current *Dietary Guidelines for Americans* (*DGA*) encourage diversifying protein intake, increasing fiber intake, and limiting consumption of red and processed meats, all of which are more consistent with a plant-forward (and lower-emission) diet. Most notably, decreasing consumption of red meat, the most carbon-intensive food, while increasing consumption of plant-based foods will prevent and mitigate diet-related chronic diseases and decrease GHG emissions.[2]

Federal Nutrition Assistance Programs

The national strategy proposes leveraging federal nutrition assistance programs, such as the National School Lunch Program and the Special Supplemental Nutrition Assistance Program for Women, Infants, and Children (WIC), to promote healthy habits. For example, the strategy includes efforts to improve the nutritional quality of school meals through an incentive program and updates to the nutrition criteria in the USDA Foods program. The administration should expand these proposals to incorporate sustainability as a criterion for foods provided under these programs as a means of both decreasing the carbon footprint of federal nutrition assistance programs and spurring the food industry to produce more sustainable products. In particular, federal nutrition assistance programs should shift toward more plant-forward offerings, which would have benefits for both climate and health.

Dietary Guidelines for Americans

The alignment between nutrition policy and climate policy should extend to the *DGA*. Published every five years by the US Department of Health and Human Services (DHHS) and the USDA, the *DGA* form the basis for nutrition standards in nutrition assistance programs across the federal government, including WIC and the National School Lunch Program. The 2015–2020 Dietary Guidelines Advisory Committee incorporated sustainability into its recommendations, concluding that dietary patterns higher in plant-based foods and lower in animal-based foods better promote health and mitigate the environmental impact of the food system.[20] The secretaries of the DHHS and USDA eliminated sustainability from the final *DGA* based on the premise that it was beyond the scope of the guidelines.

As the DHHS and USDA gear up for the 2025–2030 *DGA*, they have suggested that sustainability will be considered in a separate process. Although this decision indicates a small step in the right direction, the exclusion of sustainability from the *DGA* themselves ignores the critical role of the guidelines in federal food policy and as a model for the country. Including sustainability in the *DGA* would be a major step forward in the integration of climate policy with the federal hunger and nutrition strategy.

Federal Food Procurement

The administration can also reduce food-related GHG emissions by shifting federal food procurement to healthier, more sustainable foods. The national strategy includes an intention to expand access to healthier food environments in federal facilities by implementing and updating the Federal Food Service Guidelines (FSGs). The FSGs, issued by the Centers for Disease Control and Prevention (CDC), are evidence-based best practices for food service operations in federal facilities, such as cafeterias in federal office buildings and military facilities. Adoption of the FSGs has been voluntary; in practice, this means that they are largely ignored. The administration should issue an executive order to require implementation of the FSGs. Such an order would improve the diets of millions of federal employees, as well as people incarcerated in federal prisons, veterans receiving care from Department of Veterans Affairs hospitals, visitors to national parks, and military service members, and thereby prevent and mitigate diet-related chronic diseases.

At the same time, the CDC should update the FSGs to strengthen environmental considerations. Currently, the FSGs address some environmental factors, such as local sourcing and organic food; this should be expanded to include climate impacts, including strategies for increasing plant-based meals at federal facilities. In addition to improving the health and welfare of Americans being fed at these facilities, this approach would leverage the billions of food dollars spent by the federal government to support climate mitigation efforts. It would also be consistent with the Biden administration's separate commitment to achieve net zero procurement (inclusive of food) by 2050 through Executive Order 14057. This was a missed opportunity to put forth a specific strategy to reduce emissions associated with food procurement while also achieving co-benefits for health.

LEVERAGE SUSTAINABLE FOOD RECOVERY AND WASTE MANAGEMENT

The national strategy highlights food recovery as a method to address food insecurity. In the United States, one third of all food goes uneaten, and the production, transportation, preparation, and disposal of this wasted food contribute 8% of anthropogenic GHG emissions.[21] Food waste represents 24% and 22% of landfilled and combusted municipal solid waste, respectively.[21] When food waste is processed at a landfill, it produces methane, a potent GHG. These emissions are mitigated when food waste is processed via sustainable methods such as composting or anaerobic digestion, which also produce additional environmental benefits.[22]

Noting the high rate of food waste, the national strategy includes a commitment to developing a whole-of-government approach to reducing food loss and waste while also updating policies related to food donation. Surprisingly, the environmental effects of food waste are not mentioned. Given the outsized contribution of food waste to overall GHG emissions, this is a striking omission at odds with the Environmental Protection Agency's recent report concluding that food waste "offers an opportunity for meaningful [GHG] reductions."[21]

The administration should incorporate climate into food waste policy in two major respects. First, it should recognize that by promoting food recovery, we can reduce overall food production and thereby decrease the impact of the food system on deforestation, biodiversity loss, GHGs, and water use. Second, it should incorporate sustainability into its whole-of-government strategy for food waste by including sustainable food waste management methods in federal procurement practices, nutrition programs, and guidelines, such as the National School Lunch Program and the FSGs.

IMPROVE FOOD STORE ACCESS AND EMERGENCY FOOD AVAILABILITY

In its approach to hunger and food insecurity, the national strategy includes actions designed to improve physical access to food for the 40 million Americans, often from low-income communities and communities of color, who live in areas where grocery stores are not readily accessible. Such food access is closely tied to climate change, because extreme weather events attributable to climate change (e.g., floods and drought) are major threats to food production and access. The national strategy proposes the use of housing and community programs to increase proximity to healthy food options and directs the US Department of Transportation (DOT) to improve transportation options to and from grocery stores. Although these actions are essential to increase healthy food access in underserved communities, they should expressly incorporate climate resiliency considerations so that these communities have easy access to food even in the face of climate-related extreme weather and heat.

Similarly, the national strategy directs the USDA and the Federal Emergency Management Agency (FEMA) to improve access to emergency food, including during natural disasters, but does not mention that extreme weather events are increasing as a result of climate change and that agencies should be preparing for these changes. The national strategy should incorporate policies ensuring that food and water infrastructure are prepared to weather the effects and threats of climate change, including directing FEMA to build climate change explicitly into its food and water security planning.

IMPROVE MULTIMODAL ACCESS TO FOOD RETAIL

The national strategy includes several actions focused on using transportation and the built environment to increase access to grocery stores as well as physical activity. Transportation plays a central role in food access and accounts for 27% of US GHG emissions, the majority (57%) of which come from passenger vehicles.[23] Significant shifts away from cars and toward active transport modes such as walking, biking, and public transit are essential to achieve the administration's GHG reduction targets under the Paris Climate Agreement. At the same time, because car use is associated with decreased physical activity and increases in obesity and other chronic diseases, shifting people from cars to active transport modes improves health.[24,25]

Recognizing the health benefits of active transport, the national strategy includes several initiatives to promote active transport through DOT grants, technical support, and guidance, and it would expand the CDC's State Physical Activity and Nutrition Program to all states, including implementation of state- and community-level policies that connect pedestrians, bicycles, and public transit to daily destinations such as grocery stores. However, despite the connections between these active transport goals and the administration's broader climate goals, the environmental benefits of active transport are not mentioned in the national strategy. These actions in the national strategy should be explicitly aligned with the administration's broader climate goals, for example, by committing to improve access to grocery stores via transport modes with lower GHG emissions.

CONCLUSION

The Biden administration has recognized the urgency of the climate crisis. With the release of the National Strategy on Hunger, Nutrition, and Health, it has also begun to address the crisis of hunger and diet-related chronic disease. But it has failed to recognize how these crises are interconnected. The administration will not achieve its goals for human and planetary health unless it acts promptly to integrate climate mitigation into its strategy for hunger, nutrition, and health. AJPH

CORRESPONDENCE

Correspondence should be sent to Rachel G. Clark, JD, 950 New Hampshire Ave, Washington, DC 20052 (e-mail: rachelclark@gwu.edu). Reprints can be ordered at http://www.ajph.org by clicking the "Reprints" link.

PUBLICATION INFORMATION

Full Citation: Clark RG, Pryor S, Dietz WH. Where was climate change at the White House Conference on Hunger, Nutrition, and Health? *Am J Public Health*. 2023;113(8):844–848.

Acceptance Date: April 4, 2023.

DOI: https://doi.org/10.2105/AJPH.2023.307312

CONTRIBUTORS

R. G. Clark led the drafting of the editorial. All of the authors contributed to the conceptualization, revision, and final version of the editorial.

ACKNOWLEDGMENTS

We thank Chloe Waterman for providing helpful feedback on this editorial.

CONFLICTS OF INTEREST

William H. Dietz serves as a consultant to the Roundtable on Obesity Solutions at the National Academies of Medicine. Rachel G. Clark and Sydney Pryor have no conflicts of interest to disclose.

REFERENCES

1. The White House. President Biden sets 2030 greenhouse gas pollution reduction target aimed at creating good-paying union jobs and securing US leadership on clean energy technologies. Available at: https://www.whitehouse.gov/briefing-room/statements-releases/2021/04/22/fact-sheet-president-biden-sets-2030-greenhouse-gas-pollution-reduction-target-aimed-at-creating-good-paying-union-jobs-and-securing-u-s-leadership-on-clean-energy-technologies. Accessed November 20, 2022.
2. Willett W, Rockström J, Loken B, et al. Food in the Anthropocene: the EAT-Lancet Commission on healthy diets from sustainable food systems. *Lancet*. 2019;393(10170):447–492. https://doi.org/10.1016/S0140-6736(18)31788-4
3. Clark MA, Domingo NGG, Colgan K, et al. Global food system emissions could preclude achieving the 1.5° and 2°C climate change targets. *Science*. 2020;370(6517):705–708. https://doi.org/10.1126/science.aba7357
4. The White House. Biden-Harris administration National Strategy on Hunger, Nutrition, and Health. Available at: https://www.whitehouse.gov/wp-content/uploads/2022/09/White-House-National-Strategy-on-Hunger-Nutrition-and-Health-FINAL.pdf. Accessed November 20, 2022.
5. Swinburn BA, Kraak VI, Allender S, et al. The global syndemic of obesity, undernutrition, and climate change: the Lancet Commission report. *Lancet*. 2019;393(10173):791–846. https://doi.org/10.1016/S0140-6736(18)32822-8
6. Springmann M, Clark M, Mason-D'Croz D, et al. Options for keeping the food system within

environmental limits. *Nature.* 2018;562(7728):519–525. https://doi.org/10.1038/s41586-018-0594-0

7. Myers SS, Smith MR, Guth S, et al. Climate change and global food systems: potential impacts on food security and undernutrition. *Annu Rev Public Health.* 2017;38:259–277. https://doi.org/10.1146/annurev-publhealth-031816-044356
8. Crippa M, Solazzo E, Guizzardi D, Monforti-Ferrario F, Tubiello FN, Leip A. Food systems are responsible for a third of global anthropogenic GHG emissions. *Nat Food.* 2021;2(3):198–209. https://doi.org/10.1038/s43016-021-00225-9
9. Lesk C, Rowhani P, Ramankutty N. Influence of extreme weather disasters on global crop production. *Nature.* 2016;529(7584):84–87. https://doi.org/10.1038/nature16467
10. Vicedo-Cabrera AM, Scovronick N, Sera F, et al. The burden of heat-related mortality attributable to recent human-induced climate change. *Nat Clim Chang.* 2021;11(6):492–500. https://doi.org/10.1038/s41558-021-01058-x
11. Domingo NGG, Balasubramanian S, Thakrar SK, et al. Air quality-related health damages of food. *Proc Natl Acad Sci U S A.* 2021;118(20):e2013637118. https://doi.org/10.1073/pnas.2013637118
12. Ogden NH. Climate change and vector-borne diseases of public health significance. *FEMS Microbiol Lett.* 2017;364(19). https://doi.org/10.1093/femsle/fnx186
13. Levy K, Woster AP, Goldstein RS, Carlton EJ. Untangling the impacts of climate change on waterborne diseases: a systematic review of relationships between diarrheal diseases and temperature, rainfall, flooding, and drought. *Environ Sci Technol.* 2016;50(10):4905–4922. https://doi.org/10.1021/acs.est.5b06186
14. *Climate Change 2014: Synthesis Report. Contribution of Working Groups I, II and III to the Fifth Assessment Report of the Intergovernmental Panel on Climate Change.* Geneva, Switzerland: Intergovernmental Panel on Climate Change; 2014.
15. Rosinger AY, Bethancourt HJ, Young SL. Tap water avoidance is associated with lower food security in the United States: evidence from NHANES 2005–2018. *J Acad Nutr Diet.* 2023;123(1):29–40.e23. https://doi.org/10.1016/j.jand.2022.07.011
16. US Environmental Protection Agency. Climate change and social vulnerability in the United States: a focus on six impacts. Available at: https://www.epa.gov/cira/social-vulnerability-report. Accessed November 20, 2022.
17. Wang Y, Beydoun MA. The obesity epidemic in the United States—gender, age, socioeconomic, racial/ethnic, and geographic characteristics: a systematic review and meta-regression analysis. *Epidemiol Rev.* 2007;29(1):6–28. https://doi.org/10.1093/epirev/mxm007
18. Tilman D, Clark M. Global diets link environmental sustainability and human health. *Nature.* 2014;515(7528):518–522. https://doi.org/10.1038/nature13959
19. Hedenus F, Wirsenius S, Johansson DJA. The importance of reduced meat and dairy consumption for meeting stringent climate change targets. *Clim Change.* 2014;124(1–2):79–91. https://doi.org/10.1007/s10584-014-1104-5
20. Dietary Guidelines Advisory Committee. Scientific report of the 2015 Dietary Guidelines Advisory Committee. Available at: http://health.gov/dietaryguidelines/2015-scientific-report/PDFs/Scientific-Report-of-the-2015-Dietary-Guidelines-Advisory-Committee.pdf. Accessed November 20, 2022.
21. US Environmental Protection Agency. From farm to kitchen: the environmental impacts of US food waste. Available at: https://www.epa.gov/system/files/documents/2021-11/from-farm-to-kitchen-the-environmental-impacts-of-u.s.-food-waste_508-tagged.pdf. Accessed November 20, 2022.
22. Morris J, Scott Matthews H, Morawski C. Review and meta-analysis of 82 studies on end-of-life management methods for source separated organics. *Waste Manag.* 2013;33(3):545–551. https://doi.org/10.1016/j.wasman.2012.08.004
23. US Environmental Protection Agency. Fast facts on transportation greenhouse gas emissions. Available at: https://www.epa.gov/greenvehicles/fast-facts-transportation-greenhouse-gas-emissions. Accessed November 20, 2022.
24. Abu-Omar K, Gelius P, Messing S. Physical activity promotion in the age of climate change. *F1000Res.* 2020;9:349. https://doi.org/10.12688/f1000research.23764.2
25. Flint E, Webb E, Cummins S. Change in commute mode and body-mass index: prospective, longitudinal evidence from UK Biobank. *Lancet Public Health.* 2016;1(2):e46–e55. https://doi.org/10.1016/S2468-2667(16)30006-8

Improving Indian Health Service Vaccination Campaigns Across the Full Spectrum of Age, Clinical, and Public Health Settings

Hailey A. Baker, BS, Anna Klunk, MPH, Alec J. Calac, BS, Tamee Livermont, MPH, and Shaquita Bell, MD

ABOUT THE AUTHORS

Hailey A. Baker and Tamee Livermont are with the University of Minnesota Medical School, Minneapolis. Anna Klunk is with Philadelphia College of Medicine, Philadelphia, PA. Alec J. Calac is with the University of California San Diego School of Medicine, San Diego. Shaquita Bell is with the University of Washington and Seattle Children's Hospital, Seattle.

The Indian Health Service (IHS) is a federal agency responsible for the provision of health services to American Indians and Alaska Natives (AI/AN). Numerous treaties and laws, judicial rulings, and executive orders require that the IHS care for the physical, mental, social, and spiritual health of Native Americans enrolled in one of 574 federally recognized AI/AN tribes and villages.

One of the most significant issues faced by the IHS has been suboptimal vaccination within the AI/AN population.[1] It is well recognized that the act of vaccination, not just the availability of vaccines, is crucial to improving public health by reducing the risk of infection or severe disease course.[1,2] The IHS has long been susceptible to government shutdowns, supply chain issues, and geographic barriers that make it difficult to vaccinate geographically isolated AI/AN communities.[3] However, resource availability is not the only cause for the disparities in vaccine coverage within tribal communities; failure of federal IHS facilities to provide services and care reflective of the priorities and values of the communities they serve has only exacerbated these disparities. This has resulted in the disproportionate burden of vaccine-preventable disease within geographic AI/AN populations throughout the life course, including influenza, pneumonia, pertussis, and human papillomavirus (HPV).[1,3]

With passage of the Indian Self-Determination and Education Assistance Act of 1975, AI/AN tribes and villages obtained the ability to exercise their sovereignty over health services delivery for their communities, often resulting in tribal partnerships with academic medical centers and appropriate state and federal agencies to increase vaccine uptake. During the COVID-19 pandemic, we saw AI/AN vaccine uptake exceed that of the general population.[4] This was evidenced by efforts in communities like the Lummi Nation, where community leaders prioritized the use of traditional values, including respect for elders and collectivism, also letting community members, rather than outside agencies, shape vaccine messaging.[4]

Although these tribal-led campaigns and other public health programs have been successful in increasing community vaccination rates, the IHS now hopes to build on the success of the COVID-19 vaccination campaign and fully close all AI/AN vaccine coverage gaps with the launch of their E3 Vaccine Strategy (E3VS). E3VS emphasizes that (1) every patient at (2) every encounter should be offered (3) every recommended vaccine when appropriate.[5] However, this approach is not novel; health facilities with a community-based approach to health care have utilized this approach for decades, but a number of factors limit its effectiveness. These factors include distrust of the scientific community and vaccine development, as well as health professionals' sparse education regarding AI/AN clinical care and health beliefs, which hampers addressing the root causes of vaccine coverage disparities.[5] Thus, E3VS alone will not be enough to achieve desirable vaccine coverage in AI/AN communities. Leveraging the relationships of AI/AN community health representatives (community members who bridge health care and community spaces) may prove beneficial to IHS providers.

VACCINE HESITANCY AS A RESULT OF HISTORICAL HARMS

E3VS will ostensibly offer every recommended vaccine to unvaccinated patients

AJPH August 2023, Vol 113, No. 8

who present to a health care facility, but it does not address the variety of structural and sociocultural barriers affecting vaccine uptake. There is a complicated history between the United States and AI/AN communities, including cultural genocide, coercive sterilization, and unethical research. This history does not simply disappear when a vaccine is offered to a patient. A recent social media analysis exploring Facebook user reactions to a COVID-19 vaccine trial on a large AI/AN reservation found that 17.5% of comments were negative, with common themes being the historical and contemporary injustice against Native people.[6] Other potential contributors to vaccine hesitancy include inconsistent information regarding vaccines and vaccine-related adverse effects and lack of education provided to patients surrounding these topics by their providers.[7] For the IHS to be successful in their efforts, addressing the numerous factors influencing vaccine hesitancy through patient-centered education and shared decision-making strategies is necessary.

In addition, E3VS will feature generalized messaging to health care providers, thus missing an opportunity to speak directly to AI/AN communities regarding an important value for many: placing the needs of the community over the needs of the individual. A COVID-19 vaccination survey conducted by the Urban Indian Health Institute found that 74% of respondents willing to be vaccinated against COVID-19 believed that vaccination was a responsibility to their community. A key recommendation of the survey was to center vaccination campaigns around preservation of culture and traditions, as well as to protect loved ones, including future generations, language keepers, and the elderly.[8] Similarly, the National Indian Health Board, an AI/AN-led nonprofit, suggests including elders and tribal leaders in vaccination campaigns, ensuring that community priorities are centered.[9]

REPRESENTATION IN CLINICAL TRIALS AND VITAL STATISTICS

The long-standing underrepresentation of AI/AN individuals in clinical research trials works against efforts to promote AI/AN health equity. In a retrospective study that evaluated racial and ethnic minority populations in US-based clinical cancer trials, only 133 of 278 470 participants (0.048%) identified as AI/AN.[10]

Racial misclassification is another important aspect to consider when contextualizing AI/AN health disparities. It is estimated that up to 40% of AI/AN individuals are misclassified as non-Hispanic White on their death certificates.[11] The underreporting of AI/AN mortality rates at the local, state, and federal level may prevent targeted resourcing and timely interventions to these communities, including funds for vaccination programs.[11]

The development of the HPV vaccine is a prime example of the effects of AI/AN underrepresentation in clinical research. When the first HPV vaccine was released in 2006, it was a quadrivalent vaccine, covering high-risk HPV (hrHPV) subtypes HPV-6, HPV-11, HPV-16, and HPV-18.[12] In 2014, the nine-valent hrHPV vaccine was released, expanding coverage to HPV-31, HPV-33, HPV-45, HPV-52, and HPV-58, which were found to be the causative agents of cervical vulvovaginal, oropharyngeal, anal, and penile cancers.[13] Today, the nine-valent vaccine is estimated to cover 92% of cancers attributable to the subtypes it includes.[13] However, these subtypes do not align with the hrHPV subtype distributions found in AI/AN patients, likely because of insufficient inclusion in vaccine development.[2] When considering cancer incidence in the precision medicine era, particularly those caused by HPV, it becomes difficult to identify hrHPV subtypes driving cancer in communities inadequately represented in available clinical datasets.

HUMAN PAPILLOMAVIRUS SUBTYPE PREVALENCE

Despite the importance of vaccination for decreasing HPV-related disease, HPV vaccination rates vary in AI/AN populations, with facilities reporting variable vaccination rates compared with the general population.[2,13] Notably, AI/AN communities also have overall higher rates of hrHPV and HPV-associated cancers, with variations in cancer rates based on geographic location.[2]

AI/AN patients in recent studies were not only found to have higher rates of hrHPV compared with the national average but were also found to be affected by strains of hrHPV not prevalent in the general population. This includes HPV-51, which is not included in the nine-valent HPV vaccine.[2,13] A study of an AI/AN community in the Great Plains found that nearly one in 10 people tested for HPV were positive for HPV-51.[2] Alternatively, HPV-16, one of the strains covered in the nine-valent HPV vaccine, had the lowest prevalence in the population studied, with fewer than one in 20 people testing positive.[2]

In the case of HPV, E3VS will likely improve the HPV vaccination rate in the AI/AN population and provide optimal coverage against the nine subtypes included within the current vaccine. However, it will do little to prevent HPV-driven cancers in areas where prevalent high-risk HPV subtypes are not covered by the nine-valent HPV vaccine. To make a meaningful difference in HPV-driven cancers, the IHS should couple E3VS with other measures, including, but not limited to, communications about the importance of a yearly physical exam and Papanicolaou test administration at the time of vaccination.

RESOURCE INVESTMENT IN VACCINATION EFFORTS

Chronic underfunding of the IHS will also limit the impact of the E3VS. This makes alternative funding streams increasingly important. The Indian Health Care Improvement Act, which was permanently reauthorized in the Affordable Care Act, allowed for services delivered in IHS facilities to be billed to public programs such as Medicare and Medicaid. These revenue streams are a primary source of income for IHS and Tribal Health Programs and are vital to the procurement of supplies and services needed for facility operation, including vaccination outreach.[14]

The provision of vaccines is important but also costly. To meet the mission of the IHS, Congress must appropriate additional funds to the agency so that E3VS will not divert resources from other important health programs.

CONCLUSION

This article highlights important considerations for public health programs organized by the IHS. The United States has a moral and legal responsibility to protect and promote the health of tribal communities. To maximize benefit to all, efforts must be made to fund IHS health maintenance activities, prioritize tribal self-governance and self-determination, and make funds directly available to tribes, rather than states and other pass-through jurisdictions. Our youths, elders, language keepers, and communities at large deserve no less. AJPH

CORRESPONDENCE

Correspondence should be sent to Hailey Baker, 420 Delaware St SE, Minneapolis, MN 55455 (e-mail: bake1547@umn.edu). Reprints can be ordered at http://www.ajph.org by clicking the "Reprints" link.

PUBLICATION INFORMATION

Full Citation: Baker HA, Klunk A, Calac AJ, Livermont T, Bell S. Improving Indian health service vaccination campaigns across the full spectrum of age, clinical, and public health settings. *Am J Public Health*. 2023;113(8):849–851.

Acceptance Date: May 18, 2023.

DOI: https://doi.org/10.2105/AJPH.2023.307349

CONTRIBUTORS

H. A. Baker developed the introductory paragraphs, Vaccine Hesitancy as Result of Historical Harms and HPV Subtype Prevalence sections, as well as contributed to global edits. A. Klunk developed the introductory paragraphs and Representation in Clinical Trials and Vital Statistics section, as well as contributed to global edits. A. J. Calac developed the project and all sections, as well as contributed to global edits. T. Livermont developed the Resource Investment in Vaccination Efforts section and contributed to global edits. S. Bell contributed to global edits as well as provided critical insight to the project as a practicing physician.

ACKNOWLEDGMENTS

We acknowledge and thank the tribal nations and organizations leading vaccination efforts for American Indian and Alaska Native Peoples.

CONFLICTS OF INTEREST

The authors report no conflicts of interest.

REFERENCES

1. Nickel AJ, Puumala SE, Kharbanda AB. Vaccine-preventable hospitalizations among American Indian/Alaska Native children using the 2012 Kid's Inpatient Database. *Vaccine*. 2018;36(7):945–948. https://doi.org/10.1016/j.vaccine.2017.02.051
2. Lee NR, Winer RL, Cherne S, et al. Human papillomavirus prevalence among American Indian women of the Great Plains. *J Infect Dis*. 2019;219(6):908–915. https://doi.org/10.1093/infdis/jiy600
3. Groom AV, Cheek JE, Bryan RT. Effect of a national vaccine shortage on vaccine coverage for American Indian/Alaska Native children. *Am J Public Health*. 2006;96(4):697–701. https://doi.org/10.2105/AJPH.2004.053413
4. Silberner J. COVID-19: how Native Americans led the way in the US vaccination effort. *BMJ*. 2021;374:n2168. https://doi.org/10.1136/bmj.n2168
5. Indian Health Service. Indian Health Service E3 Vaccine Strategy. 2022. Available at: https://www.ihs.gov/sites/nptc/themes/responsive2017/display_objects/documents/e3vaccinestrategy/IHS-E3-Vaccine-Strategy_DOCUMENT.pdf. Accessed November 5, 2022.
6. Calac AJ, Bardier C, Cai M, Mackey TK. Examining Facebook community reaction to a COVID-19 vaccine trial on the Navajo Nation. *Am J Public Health*. 2021;111(8):1428–1430. https://doi.org/10.2105/AJPH.2021.306202
7. Jim C, Wai-Yin Lee J, Groom A, Espey D. Human papillomavirus vaccination practices among providers in Indian Health Service, tribal and urban Indian healthcare facilities. *J Womens Health (Larchmt)*. 2012;21(4):372–378. https://doi.org/10.1089/jwh.2011.3417
8. Urban Indian Health Institute. Strengthening vaccine efforts in Indian Country. Available at: https://www.uihi.org/projects/strengthening-vaccine-efforts-in-indian-country. Accessed November 23, 2022.
9. National Indian Health Board. Vaccine confidence and uptake strategies for tribal communities. Available at: https://www.nihb.org/covid-19/wp-content/uploads/2022/07/COVID-19-Vaccine-Confidence-and-Uptake-Strategies.pdf. Accessed November 23, 2022.
10. Cayatineto H, Clyde C, Yazzie G, Selassie G, de Soto J. The systemic exclusion of Native Americans from cancer clinical trials. *J Med Res Health Sci*. 2021;4(7):1396–1404. https://doi.org/10.52845/JMRHS/2021-4-8-4
11. Richardson G. Sidebar: impact of racial misclassification of health data on American Indians in North Carolina. *N C Med J*. 2021;82(6):399–400. https://doi.org/10.18043/ncm.82.6.399
12. Centers for Disease Control and Prevention. Use of 9-valent human papillomavirus (HPV) vaccine: updated HPV vaccination recommendations of the Advisory Committee on Immunization Practices. 2015. Available at: https://www.cdc.gov/mmwr/preview/mmwrhtml/mm6411a3.htm#:~:text=9%2Dvalent%20HPV%20vaccine%20(9vHPV,45%2C%2052%2C%20and%2058. Accessed May 14, 2023.
13. Senkomago V, Henley SJ, Thomas CC, Mix JM, Markowitz LE, Saraiya M. Human papillomavirus–attributable cancers—United States, 2012–2016. *MMWR Morb Mortal Wkly Rep*. 2019;68(33):724–728. https://doi.org/10.15585/mmwr.mm6833a3
14. Rosenberg M. Indian Health Service: information on third-party collections and processes to procure supplies and services. US Government Accountability Office. March 10, 2022. Available at: https://www.gao.gov/products/gao-22-104742. Accessed December 5, 2022.

Why Are We Going Backward? Barriers to Disaggregated Racial Information in Federal Data Sets

Armaan Jamal, BS, Malathi Srinivasan, MD, Gloria Kim, MD, Robert J. Huang, MD, MS, and Latha Palaniappan, MD, MS

ABOUT THE AUTHORS

All authors are with the Stanford Center for Asian Health Research and Education, Stanford University School of Medicine, Stanford, CA. Armaan Jamal is also with the Department of Medicine, Johns Hopkins University School of Medicine, Baltimore, MD. Malathi Srinivasan is also with the Division of Primary Care and Population Health, Stanford University School of Medicine. Gloria Kim is also with the Division of Cardiovascular Medicine, Stanford University School of Medicine. Robert J. Huang is also with the Division of Gastroenterology and Hepatology, Stanford University School of Medicine. Latha Palaniappan is also with the Division of Cardiovascular Medicine, Stanford University School of Medicine.

AJPH August 2023, Vol 113, No. 8

See also Kapadia, p. 839.

Approximately 7% of the United States population is composed of Asian American, Native Hawaiian, and Pacific Islander (AANHPI) communities. Though often aggregated in research studies, AANHPI populations in the United States are diverse, originating from 50 countries and speaking more than 100 languages. Aggregation may mask significant disparities between AANHPI subgroups, including the prevalence of chronic conditions and access to care.[1] Disaggregation of health data for AANHPI populations has been a priority of the US Department of Health and Human Services (HHS) for more than 20 years, and collection of disaggregated AANHPI data in US federal health data sets has increased over that time.[1] However, a large gap remains between the collection of these data and their practical and meaningful use for public health research, mainly because of the burdens placed on researchers to access these data.

BARRIERS IN ACCESSING DISAGGREGATED DATA

Federal data sets collecting disaggregated AANHPI data often contain small sample sizes with respect to subgroups. Restrictions to ensure robust protection of security and confidentiality must be in place; however, in certain cases, these restrictions go beyond what is reasonable and necessary to protect privacy. They are excessively burdensome and serve to dissuade researchers from using these data. For example, to use disaggregated data from the National Center for Health Statistics, an individual must first submit, revise, and have accepted an application—a complex review process that can take months to years. Once the application is approved, the researcher must submit statistical code and shell tables for approval.[2,3] The researcher must then physically travel to one of 33 Research Data Centers in the United States to extract data and perform analysis under direct supervision, paying for each day of data access, with no future access to clarify findings.

Hypothesis-driven secondary data analysis is a common method for answering clinically relevant questions when relationships between variables are well understood. However, exploring a data set informed by clinical and public health experiences identifies new gaps and hypotheses—especially when new variables are examined, such as race or factors influenced by new public health events. With new data sets, specific cutpoints for variables may be difficult to make without data exploration. In addition, requiring travel to one of the few data centers dispersed throughout the United States decreases the feasibility of this option for many researchers with financial constraints. Other barriers involve long processing times and fees that may exceed \$10 000.[2,3] Processing times vary depending on the data collection agency but may range from a few months to years. By then, data are less relevant for public health, the findings stale, and journals less likely to publish "old news." These restrictions further amplify existing disparities. For example, during the COVID-19 pandemic, federal sites only admitted US citizens.[4]

Such barriers to access may partially explain the limited literature on disaggregated AANHPI populations published from National Center for Health Statistics data sources. Similar barriers exist with data sets collected by the Agency for Healthcare Research and

Quality, the Centers for Medicare and Medicaid Services, the Health Resources and Services Administration, and the Substance Abuse and Mental Health Services Administration.[5–7] Moreover, some federal data sets that had previously allowed public access to disaggregated data, such as the National Health Interview Survey (NHIS), have recently restricted access.[8]

Table 1 presents a summary of health surveys and nonsurvey data collected by HHS (e.g., National Vital Statistics) that contain disaggregated AANHPI data from years 2011 to 2021, building on work by

TABLE 1— Public Availability of Disaggregated Data on Asian Americans, Native Hawaiians, and Pacific Islanders in the US Department of Health and Human Services Patient Surveys and Collected Data, 2011–2021

Survey (Agency)	Year Disaggregated AANHPI Data Collection Began	Disaggregated Data Publicly Available?	Data That Are Available to Public
Medical Expenditure Panel Survey (AHRQ)	2011 (Asian American), 2012 (NH/PI)	Yes	Asian Indian, Chinese, Filipino, and other Asians and NH/PI
Behavioral Risk Factor Surveillance System (CDC)	2013	No	"Asians" and "NH/PI" separate categories
National Health and Nutrition Examination Survey (CDC)	2011	No	"Asians" available as a single category and NH/PI aggregated with other races and multiple races as "other races, including multiracial"
National Health Interview Survey (CDC)	2011	Yes	Asian Indian, Filipino, Chinese, and other Asian available through 2018. After 2018, Asians, and NH/PI aggregated as "Asians"
Native Hawaiian and Pacific Islander National Health Interview Survey (CDC)	2014	Yes	Asian Indian, Filipino, Chinese, other Asian and NH/PI. Disaggregated NH/PI groups available through the restricted data set
National Immunization Survey (CDC)	2015	No	"Asians" and "NH/PI" separate categories
National Survey of Children's Health (CDC 2011–2012; HRSA 2016–2021)	2016	No	"Asians" and "NH/PI" separate categories
National Survey of Family Growth (CDC)	2013	No	AANHPI communities categorized as "Other"
National Vital Statistics Mortality Data (CDC)	2011	Yes	Chinese, Japanese, Hawaiian, Filipino, Asian Indian, Korean, Samoan, Vietnamese, Guamanian, and other Asian or Pacific Islanders
National Vital Statistics Birth Record Data (CDC)	2011	Yes	Chinese, Japanese, Hawaiian, Filipino, Asian Indian, Korean, Samoan, Vietnamese, Guamanian, and other Asian or Pacific Islanders
CAHPS for Accountable Care Organizations Participating in Medicare Initiatives (CMS)	2013	No	"Asians" and "NH/PI" separate categories
CAHPS for Merit-Based Incentive Payment System (CMS)	2016	No	"Asians" and "NH/PI" separate categories
Health Outcomes Survey (CMS)	2013	No	"Asians" and "NH/PI" separate categories
Home and Community Based CAHPS (CMS)	2017	No	"Asians" and "NH/PI" separate categories
In-Center Hemodialysis CAHPS (CMS)	2015	No	"Asians" and "NH/PI" separate categories
Medicare Current Beneficiary Survey (CMS)	2015	No	"Asians" and "NH/PI" separate categories
Nationwide Adult Medicaid CAHPS (CMS)	2014	No	"Asians" and "NH/PI" separate categories
Outpatient and Ambulatory Surgery CAHPS (CMS)	2016	No	"Asians" and "NH/PI" separate categories
National Survey on Drug Use and Health (SAMHSA)	2011 (Asian American), 2013 (NH/PI)	No	"Asians" and "NH/PI" separate categories

Note. AANHPI = Asian American, Native Hawaiian, or Pacific Islander; AHRQ = Agency for Healthcare Research and Quality; CAHPS = Consumer Assessment of Healthcare Provider and Systems; CDC = Centers for Disease Control and Prevention; CMS = Centers for Medicare and Medicaid Services; HRSA = Health Resources and Services Administration; NH/PI = Native Hawaiian or Pacific Islander; SAMHSA = Substance Abuse and Mental Health Services Administration.

Nguyen et al.[1] Our summary includes the year disaggregated data collection began, whether disaggregated data are available publicly, and the type of data that are publicly available. Additional information on the steps to access and the estimated cost to acquire data can be found in Table A (available as a supplement to the online version of this article at https://ajph.org).

We found that most federal data sets collected by HHS agencies do not make disaggregated AANHPI data publicly available. Of our sample of 19 federal data sets, only five make this data public: the NHIS, the Native Hawaiian and Pacific Islander NHIS, the Medical Expenditure Panel Survey, and the mortality and birth records data from the National Vital Statistics System. Of these, only the National Vital Statistics System data sets allow public access to the full spectrum of disaggregated race codes.[9]

Legislative, logistical, and financial barriers exist in accessing restricted AANHPI data, which vary by data set. Out of the 19 data sets, 16 allowed restricted access to disaggregated AANHPI data and all 16 required the submission of an application and research proposal to begin access. Eight of the 16 required prior approval of statistical code, travel to a data center, and submission of statistical output for review. The minimum costs of data access ranged from $600 to more than $6750; costs may escalate steeply based on the number of years of data requested, proposal amendments, project renewals, and the cost of obtaining Special Sworn Status (individuals are sworn for life to protect the data of the Census Bureau as they access restricted data).[5,10] Notably, these estimates do not include travel costs to data centers.

OPPORTUNITIES TO EXPAND AVAILABILITY OF DISAGGREGATED DATA

We commend federal health agencies for recognizing the importance of disaggregated racial health data collection. We affirm and respect the cardinal importance of privacy and confidentiality in health data. However, there must be reasonable balance between security and usability, as the goals of collecting disaggregated data are to improve human health and reduce health disparities. We propose critical steps to make AANHPI data available to investigators, in an ethical and useful manner, to reduce AANHPI health disparities:

1. Develop data use agreements with investigators similar to agreements used for other sensitive medical data sets, such as cancer registries. Such agreements allow vetted investigators access to the data set, impose significant penalties for misuse, and outline security measures to which the institution and investigators must adhere. Once approved, cancer registries like the National Cancer Institute Surveillance, Epidemiology, and End Results (SEER) Program allow users data access from their own device through the SEER*Stat software by signing a data use agreement.[11] Federal data sets can employ this approach.
2. Reduce financial barriers to utilize federally collected data by collaborating with institutions that can subsidize access and processing costs for researchers. Currently, an investigator would need significant grant funding to answer even a few questions in a specific area.
3. Increase overall sampling of AANHPI populations to minimize data suppression. This may be improved through culturally sensitive community outreach and language assistance. The National Health and Nutrition Examination Survey has used such methods to oversample AANHPI populations since 2011.[12]
4. Oversample areas with high concentrations of AANHPI populations to increase sample size. This may be assisted by endorsement from local organizations and community leaders, and promotion in media, newsletters, and meetings, as demonstrated by the National Health and Nutrition Examination Survey.[12]
5. Standardize data collection between disparate federal agencies to collect sufficient sample sizes of disaggregated AANHPI communities and minimize data suppression within each agency.
6. Increase funding for disaggregated AANHPI population health survey research. Funding for Latinx and African American health has increased over the past few decades.

The AANHPI community is not a monolith, and many AANHPI communities face a disproportionate share of illness burden. By increasing thoughtful access to disaggregated health data in our national data sets, we can close the sizable gap in AANHPI population health disparities and use these findings to improve human health more precisely. AJPH

CORRESPONDENCE

Correspondence should be sent to Armaan Jamal, 720 Rutland Ave, Ross Research Building Room 1064, Baltimore, MD 21205 (e-mail: ajamal6@stanford.edu). Reprints can be ordered at https://ajph.org by clicking the "Reprints" link.

PUBLICATION INFORMATION

Full Citation: Jamal A, Srinivasan M, Kim G, Huang RJ, Palaniappan L. Why are we going backward? barriers to disaggregated racial information in federal data sets. *Am J Public Health*. 2023;113(8): 852–855.

Acceptance Date: May 12, 2023.

DOI: https://doi.org/10.2105/AJPH.2023.307339

CONTRIBUTORS

All authors sufficiently contributed to the conceptualization, design, drafting, and revision of content of this opinion editorial and approved the final version for publication.

CONFLICTS OF INTEREST

The authors have no potential or actual conflicts of interest to disclose.

REFERENCES

1. Nguyen KH, Lew KP, Trivedi AN. Trends in collection of disaggregated Asian American, Native Hawaiian, and Pacific Islander data: opportunities in federal health surveys. *Am J Public Health*. 2022;112(10):1429–1435. https://doi.org/10.2105/AJPH.2022.306969
2. National Center for Health Statistics. Location of access. November 14, 2021. Available at: https://www.cdc.gov/rdc/b2accessmod/ACs200.htm. Accessed October 16, 2022.
3. National Center for Health Statistics. Accessing restricted data. August 14, 2020. Available at: https://www.cdc.gov/rdc/leftbrch/UseRestricdt.htm. Accessed December 10, 2022.
4. Research Data Assistance Center. CMS non-US based researcher policy. Available at: https://resdac.org/articles/cms-non-us-based-researcher-policy. Accessed December 10, 2022.
5. Agency for Healthcare Research and Quality. Restricted data files available at the Data Centers. Available at: https://meps.ahrq.gov/data_stats/onsite_datacenter.jsp. Accessed October 16, 2022.
6. Centers for Medicare and Medicaid Services. Limited data set (LDS) files. Available at: https://www.cms.gov/Research-Statistics-Data-and-Systems/Files-for-Order/Data-Disclosures-Data-Agreements/DUA_-_NewLDS. Accessed October 16, 2022.
7. National Center for Health Statistics. Other restricted-use data available through the RDC. June 23, 2022. Available at: https://www.cdc.gov/rdc/b1datatype/Dt130.htm Accessed October 16, 2022.
8. National Center for Health Statistics. National Health Interview Survey—2019 NHIS. April 5, 2021. Available at: https://www.cdc.gov/nchs/nhis/2019nhis.htm. Accessed October 31, 2022.
9. National Center for Health Statistics. Vital Statistics online data portal. October 27, 2022. Available at: https://www.cdc.gov/nchs/data_access/vitalstatsonline.htm. Accessed December 10, 2022.
10. National Center for Health Statistics. Federal statistical RDC. Available at: https://www.cdc.gov/rdc/b2accessmod/ACs220.htm. Accessed May 25, 2023.
11. National Cancer Institute, Surveillance, Epidemiology, and End Results Program. How to request access to SEER Data. Available at: https://seer.cancer.gov/data/access.html. Accessed May 3, 2023.
12. Paulose-Ram R, Burt V, Broitman L, Ahluwalia N. Overview of Asian American data collection, release, and analysis: National Health and Nutrition Examination Survey 2011–2018. *Am J Public Health*. 2017;107(6):916–921. https://doi.org/10.2105/AJPH.2017.303815

Addressing Commercial Determinants to End High Tobacco Dependence Among Adolescents

Armando Peruga, MD, DrPH, and Esteve Fernández, MD, PhD

ABOUT THE AUTHORS

Armando Peruga and Esteve Fernández are with the Tobacco Control Unit, Cancer Prevention and Control Programme, Institut Català d'Oncologia/Institut d'Investigació Biomèdica de Bellvitge (ICO/IDIBELL), L'Hospitalet de Llobregat, Barcelona, Spain. Armando Peruga is also with the Center for Epidemiology and Health Policies, School of Medicine Clínica Alemana, Universidad del Desarrollo, Región Metropolitana, Chile. Esteve Fernández is also with the Center for Biomedical Research in Respiratory Diseases, Instituto de Salud Carlos III, Madrid, Spain.

See also Mehrotra et al., p. 859, and Yang et al., p. 861.

AJPH August 2023, Vol 113, No. 8

For 25 years, the US Centers for Disease Control and Prevention and the World Health Organization (WHO) have promoted the Global Youth Tobacco Survey (GYTS). This worldwide collaborative surveillance initiative involves multiple governments and nongovernmental organizations. The GYTS is designed to enhance the capacity of countries to monitor tobacco use among youths and to assess the implementation of tobacco prevention and control programs. Today, 166 countries and 16 territories have conducted the GYTS at least once, and 135 countries and nine territories at least twice (https://bit.ly/3phQNly). Based on these surveys, it is estimated that 17.9% (16.1%–19.6%) of boys aged 13 to 15 years and 11.5% (10.5%–12.4%) of girls the same age currently use tobacco products worldwide.[1] This amounts to 38 million users (https://bit.ly/3VFm4BF).

HIGH LEVELS OF TOBACCO DEPENDENCE AT AN EARLY AGE

In this issue of *AJPH*, Yang et al. (p. 861) provide for the first time, to our knowledge, a sense of the dependence that tobacco creates among current tobacco users in their early adolescence. This study's figures are staggering: 40% of the users are already dependent on nicotine from tobacco products before their 17th birthday. Hence, they have a high chance of continuing tobacco use into their late adolescence and early adulthood.

Although not unexpected, one key finding of this study is the significant gender differences in the countries' prevalences of tobacco dependence. Although globally boys have a higher statistically significant prevalence of dependence than girls (40.6% vs 33.1%), this male dominance is only evident in the Eastern Mediterranean and Southeast Asia regions. Tobacco dependence is higher among girls than boys in Europe and the Americas, although the difference is not statistically significant in the latter region. Of the 125 jurisdictions analyzed in this study, 23 presented a higher prevalence of tobacco dependence among girls than boys. This fact is a reminder that gender, either acting alone or through its intersection with other determinants of health, is a crucial driver of tobacco use and its related morbidity and mortality. When gender is considered in the design of tobacco control policies, when addressing not only women and girls but also men, boys, and masculinities, there is a more beneficial impact than when gender is overlooked.[2]

PREDICTORS OF TOBACCO DEPENDENCE

The predictors of tobacco dependence are varied. Perhaps younger age when starting to smoke is associated with higher levels of dependence, the same way that it is associated with a higher number of cigarettes smoked[3] and higher nicotine dependence in adulthood.[4] Yang et al. analyze several variables as predictors of tobacco dependence. Two normative variables, parental and close-friend smoking, are positively associated with tobacco dependence among adolescents currently using tobacco. A systematic review and meta-analysis of prospective cohort studies found that adolescents' smoking initiation odds doubled when they had parents or close friends who smoke.[5] The review did not see the same association for smoking escalation once having initiated tobacco use. This study, however, suggests that smoking in social networks close to adolescents is also a predictor of their tobacco dependence once they become tobacco users. Therefore, targeting these close social networks is essential when reducing tobacco dependence among adolescents.

The study also shows that exposure to secondhand tobacco smoke (SHS), as well as to advertising and promoting tobacco products, increases the odds of tobacco dependence among adolescents once they have started using tobacco. This association is probably shared with the constellation of factors that increase demand for tobacco products, of which the lack of protection from exposure to SHS and advertising and promoting tobacco products are part. Protecting youths from exposure to SHS, advertising, and promotion of tobacco products, as well as from critical factors that increase demand for tobacco products, such as product affordability, requires governmental action against the tobacco industry's and its allies' commercial interests.

There is evidence that comprehensive tobacco control programs decrease the prevalence of tobacco use among adults and young people by reducing consumption and increasing quitting (https://bit.ly/3nyGm2T). It has been known for a long time that jurisdictions with more extensive tobacco control policies had significantly lower youth smoking rates.[6] The results of the Yang et al. study hint that this may also be the case for the prevalence of tobacco dependence.

STRATEGIES TO END HIGH TOBACCO DEPENDENCE AMONG ADOLESCENTS

The study's results beg the question of what to do to reduce tobacco use and dependence among youths. Behavioral approaches have been recommended to reduce the initiation and scalation of adolescent tobacco use. Behavioral interventions are aimed at educating young people on the risks of tobacco and encouraging alternative behaviors to mitigate those risks. Approaches to change social norms have also been recommended, given the influence of smoking among the close social networks of adolescents also detected in the Yang et al. study. However, the precise intervention parameters to maximize the strength of these interventions among specific groups of adolescents are still a matter of research. Also, their population reach is limited, not least by the cost of scaling up these interventions to achieve a large population impact. This limitation is of particular concern in the Global South.

A strategy to reduce the initiation and scalation of adolescent tobacco use needs to be multipronged, and there is evidence of effective measures for each approach. However, behavioral health interventions targeted at changing individual behavior have been less effective than changing government policies and business environments that shape individual choices.[7] Governmental policy changes require multiple actions by multiple stakeholders to create an enabling environment to curb the tobacco epidemic.

Governmental policies to regulate the market and nonmarket business practices are key to creating an enabling environment, including prominently fiscal policy strategies to decrease the affordability of tobacco products. Governmental policies to reduce tobacco use and dependence in adolescents should be directed at reducing the demand and supply of tobacco products. Increasing the demand and supply of novel emerging nicotine products is an inadequate alternative, at least while their alleged long-term comparative health benefits need to be clarified and sanctioned by adequate regulatory agencies.[8] They are not a viable alternative while population and individual dual use of conventional tobacco products and novel emerging nicotine products coexist. The same industry has the levers to manipulate the demand and supply of both types of products as they have done during the last century.

Alas, the tobacco industry continues to be the main barrier to tobacco control. The tobacco industry's and its allies' interference is the most common barrier that parties to the WHO Framework Convention Tobacco Control face in implementing the Convention.[9] The tobacco industry is notorious for its callous attempt to exploit gender norms and influence national and international policies to advance its profits, disregarding its products' devastating health, social, environmental, and economic consequences. We suspect that many countries are already caught between the struggle to enhance democratic freedoms and human rights to protect their youths from tobacco dependence and the commercial interests of the tobacco industry and its allies. As WHO Director-General Tedros Adhanom Ghebreyesus writes, "public health cannot progress without action on the commercial determinants of health."[10] AJPH

CORRESPONDENCE

Correspondence should be sent to Armando Peruga, MD, DrPH, ICO, Unitat de Control del Tabac, Avinguda de la Granvia de l'Hospitalet, 199-203, 08908 L'Hospitalet de Llobregat, Barcelona, España (e-mail: aperuga@idibell.cat). Reprints can be ordered at https://ajph.org by clicking the "Reprints" link.

PUBLICATION INFORMATION

Full Citation: Peruga A, Fernández E. Addressing commercial determinants to end high tobacco dependence among adolescents. *Am J Public Health*. 2023;113(8):856–858.

Acceptance Date: April 28, 2023.

DOI: https://doi.org/10.2105/AJPH.2023.307330

CONTRIBUTORS

A. Peruga contributed to conceptualization, writing the original draft, and review and editing of the article. E. Fernández contributed to conceptualization and review and editing of the article.

ACKNOWLEDGMENTS

No specific funding was used to write this article. However, we acknowledge the funding of the Tobacco Control Unit at ICO by the Ministry of Research and Universities of the Government of Catalonia (grant 2021SGR00906).

CONFLICTS OF INTEREST

The authors have no conflicts of interest to declare.

REFERENCES

1. Ma C, Xi B, Li Z, et al. Prevalence and trends in tobacco use among adolescents aged 13–15 years in 143 countries, 1999–2018: findings from the Global Youth Tobacco Surveys. *Lancet Child Adolesc Health*. 2021;5(4):245–255. https://doi.org/10.1016/S2352-4642(20)30390-4
2. Hawkes S, Buse K, Soon S-Y. Gender-responsive tobacco control: evidence and options for policies and programmes. World Health Organization Framework Convention on Tobacco Control Secretariat. 2018. Available at: https://fctc.who.int/publications/m/item/gender-responsive-tobacco-control-evidence-and-options-for-policies-and-programmes. Accessed April 10, 2023.
3. Fernandez E, Schiaffino A, La Vecchia C, et al. Age at starting smoking and number of cigarettes smoked in Catalonia, Spain. *Prev Med*. 1999;28(4):361–366. https://doi.org/10.1006/pmed.1998.0433
4. John U, Meyer C, Hapke U, Rumpf HJ. Nicotine dependence and lifetime amount of smoking in a population sample. *Eur J Public Health*. 2004;14(2):182–185. https://doi.org/10.1093/eurpub/14.2.182
5. East K, McNeill A, Thrasher JF, Hitchman SC. Social norms as a predictor of smoking uptake among youth: a systematic review, meta-analysis and meta-regression of prospective cohort studies. *Addiction*. 2021;116(11):2953–2967. https://doi.org/10.1111/add.15427
6. Luke DA. State youth-access tobacco control policies and youth smoking behavior in the United States. *Am J Prev Med*. 2000;19(3):180–187. https://doi.org/10.1016/S0749-3797(00)00196-3
7. Lee K, Freudenberg N. Public health roles in addressing commercial determinants of health. *Annu Rev Public Health*. 2022;43(1):375–395. https://doi.org/10.1146/annurev-publhealth-052220-020447
8. Banks E, Yazidjoglou A, Brown S, et al. Electronic cigarettes and health outcomes: umbrella and systematic review of the global evidence. *Med J Aust*. 2023;218(6):267–275. https://doi.org/10.5694/mja2.51890
9. Convention Secretariat. *2021 Global Progress Report on Implementation of the WHO Framework Convention on Tobacco Control*. World Health Organization Framework Convention on Tobacco Control. 2022. Available at: https://fctc.who.int/publications/i/item/9789240041769. Accessed April 11, 2023.
10. Ghebreyesus TA. Achieving health for all requires action on the economic and commercial determinants of health. *Lancet*. 2023;401(10383):1137–1139. https://doi.org/10.1016/S0140-6736(23)00574-3

Tobacco Dependence in Adolescents: What Lies Ahead?

Ravi Mehrotra, MD, DPhil, Kavita Yadav, BDS, MPH, and Kamran Siddiqi, MBBS, MRCP, PhD, MPH

ABOUT THE AUTHORS

Ravi Mehrotra is an adjunct professor at Emory University, Atlanta, GA. Kavita Yadav is a research fellow at George Institute for Global Health, New Delhi, India. Kamran Siddiqi is a professor in global public health, University of York, York, United Kingdom.

See also Peruga and Fernández, p. 856, and Yang et al., p. 861.

The article by Yang et al. in this issue of *AJPH* (p. 861) reports the global prevalence of tobacco dependence as 38.4% (95% confidence interval [CI] = 34.0, 42.7) among adolescents who currently smoke tobacco. They conclude that exposure to secondhand smoke, parental smoking, closest friends smoking, tobacco advertisement exposure, and being offered free tobacco products were all positively associated with tobacco dependence among adolescents.

Tobacco is among the addictive substances most commonly consumed by adolescents and young adults, second only to alcohol.[1] It has been found that nine of 10 children initiate smoking before they reach 18 years of age and often continue to smoke.[2] Globally, at least 43.8 million adolescents aged 13 to 15 years use some form of tobacco. Southeast Asia has the largest number of child tobacco users aged 13 to 15 years (14.8 million, or 34% of the global total for this age group).[3] Extensive tobacco use among youths has been found to increase the numbers of serious oral and systemic diseases.[4] The most recent global prevalence of cigarette smoking was 11.3% (95% CI = 10.3, 12.3) among boys and 6.1% (95% CI = 5.6, 6.6) among girls.[5] Therefore, it is important to understand adolescent tobacco dependence and its associated factors so that the problem of tobacco addiction in adults can be halted right where it starts: in adolescence.

The use of tobacco by parents, as well as secondhand smoke exposure, has been found to be strongly associated with tobacco use in young adolescents.[6] The article by Yang et al. strengthens the existing literature on tobacco use in adolescents and its associated factors.

When it comes to addressing tobacco dependence, prevention and cessation go hand in hand. Until now, most tobacco cessation efforts have primarily focused on adults, emphasizing regular smokers. The study by Yang et al. highlights the necessity of tailor-made tobacco control strategies and measures in light of the prevalence of tobacco dependence among adolescents who currently smoke tobacco in different countries and World Bank regions. The establishment of unified diagnostic criteria for tobacco dependence among adolescents for early identification and timely treatment, especially in countries with high prevalence, would be helpful.

POINTS TO PONDER

Yang et al. provide valuable insights into tobacco dependence among adolescents worldwide and underscore the importance of addressing the social, environmental, and economic factors that contribute to tobacco use. This is of great value, as the same factors that predispose adolescents to take up smoking are also contributing to making them tobacco dependent. The authors acknowledge the limitation that their study relies on self-reported data, which may be subject to recall and social desirability biases. In addition, questions related to tobacco dependence did not involve smokeless tobacco, which may lead to an underestimation of the extent of overall tobacco dependence. Smokeless tobacco is the predominant form of tobacco use among adolescents in South Asia.[7] Gender is another significant construct influencing smoking initiation, and concerted research efforts are required to understand this.[8]

RECOMMENDATIONS

The problem of tobacco dependence in youths is multifaceted and hence needs a multipronged approach for its solution. Individual factors, family dynamics, and the community play an important role.

Better enforcement of the existing rules to prevent sales of tobacco to and by minors will help to deter early exposure to tobacco and would be helpful in the long run. Tobacco cessation programs should be aimed at adolescents with tobacco dependence and cater to their psychological needs. An increased

AJPH August 2023, Vol 113, No. 8

push for in-depth research is needed to understand gender roles in tobacco dependence and cessation.

Other approaches may include restricting access to tobacco, limiting its marketing, and conducting media campaigns that focus on the harmful effects of tobacco use. Improving tobacco prevention and cessation awareness activities at the school level by creating "youth ambassadors" or "champions" might help influence impressionable young minds. Using social media to cater to the young population to spread awareness (e.g., influencers advocating for quitting tobacco) can also change adolescents' attitudes. By refusing to support tobacco use or appear in surrogate advertisements, prominent personalities such as movie stars and athletes could positively affect both adolescents and adults. Apart from these, preventing tobacco sales to adolescents would help deter early exposure to tobacco and be beneficial in the long run. Tobacco cessation programs are aimed at adolescents and cater to their psychological needs. An increased push for in-depth research is needed to understand gender roles in tobacco dependence and cessation. Prevention and cessation programs must be designed to address other tobacco products besides cigarettes. Health care professionals have key responsibilities in preventing tobacco use among youths and their families, and they need to know more about effective smoking prevention and cessation strategies. Clinicians need to integrate tobacco counseling into health assessments of teenagers and be aware of the roles that families, communities, and governments can play in promoting tobacco-free environments.[9]

Parents' refraining from tobacco use would also set an example that adolescents can look up to. As they say, any nation's greatest wealth and strength is its youths. The future of a nation lies in the hands of its posterity. If we want to ensure a healthy future for our world, we first need to strengthen and empower our young population, and prevention of tobacco use is one of the best ways to ensure that. AJPH

CORRESPONDENCE

Correspondence should be sent to Ravi Mehrotra, MD, DPhil, FRCPath, Adjunct Professor, Emory University, 1518 Clifton Rd, Atlanta, GA 30322 (e-mail: ravi.mehrotra@emory.edu). Reprints can be ordered at http://www.ajph.org by clicking the "Reprints" link.

PUBLICATION INFORMATION

Full Citation: Mehrotra R, Yadav K, Siddiqi K. Tobacco dependence in adolescents: what lies ahead? *Am J Public Health*. 2023;113(8):859–860.

Acceptance Date: May 16, 2023.

DOI: https://doi.org/10.2105/AJPH.2023.307342

CONTRIBUTORS

R. Mehrotra conceptualized the article and provided overall supervision and guidance. K. Yadav wrote and edited the first draft, and K. Siddiqi critically reviewed it.

CONFLICTS OF INTEREST

The authors have no conflicts of interest to report.

REFERENCES

1. Currie C, Zanotti C, Morgan A, et al. Social determinants of health and well-being among young people: Health Behaviour in School-Aged Children (HBSC) Study. International report from the 2009/2010 survey. World Health Organization Regional Office for Europe. 2012. Available at: https://www.who.int/europe/initiatives/health-behaviour-in-school-aged-children-(hbsc)-study. Accessed May 4, 2023.
2. US National Center for Chronic Disease Prevention and Health Promotion, Office on Smoking and Health. The health consequences of smoking—50 years of progress: a report of the surgeon general. 2014. Available at: https://www.ncbi.nlm.nih.gov/books/NBK179276. Accessed May 4, 2023.
3. WHO global report on trends in prevalence of tobacco use 2000–2025, 3rd ed. World Health Organization. Available at: https://www.who.int/publications-detail-redirect/who-global-report-on-trends-in-prevalence-of-tobacco-use-2000-2025-third-edition. Accessed May 4, 2023.
4. Nazir MA, Al-Ansari A, Abbasi N, Almas K. Global prevalence of tobacco use in adolescents and its adverse oral health consequences. *Open Access Maced J Med Sci*. 2019;7(21):3659–3666. https://doi.org/10.3889/oamjms.2019.542
5. Ma C, Xi B, Li Z, et al. Prevalence and trends in tobacco use among adolescents aged 13–15 years in 143 countries, 1999–2018: findings from the Global Youth Tobacco Surveys. *Lancet Child Adolesc Health*. 2021;5(4):245–255. https://doi.org/10.1016/S2352-4642(20)30390-4
6. Xi B, Liang Y, Liu Y, et al. Tobacco use and second-hand smoke exposure in young adolescents aged 12–15 years: data from 68 low-income and middle-income countries. *Lancet Glob Health*. 2016;4(11):e795–e805. https://doi.org/10.1016/S2214-109X(16)30187-5
7. Mishu MP, Siddiqui F, Shukla R, Kanaan M, Dogar O, Siddiqi K. Predictors of cigarette smoking, smokeless tobacco consumption, and use of both forms in adolescents in South Asia: a secondary analysis of the Global Youth Tobacco Surveys. *Nicotine Tob Res*. 2021;23(6):956–965. https://doi.org/10.1093/ntr/ntaa202
8. Mehrotra R, Yadav A, Sinha DN, et al. Smokeless tobacco control in 180 countries across the globe: call to action for full implementation of WHO FCTC measures. *Lancet Oncol*. 2019;20(4):e208–e217. https://doi.org/10.1016/S1470-2045(19)30084-1
9. National Cancer Institute. Changing adolescent smoking prevalence. Available at: https://cancercontrol.cancer.gov/sites/default/files/2020-08/m14_complete.pdf. Accessed May 4, 2023.

Prevalence of and Factors Associated With Tobacco Dependence Among Adolescents Aged 12–16 Years Who Were Currently Smoking Tobacco in 125 Countries or Territories, 2012–2019

Hui Yang, Chuanwei Ma, MS, Min Zhao, MD, and Bo Xi, MD

See also Peruga and Fernández, p. 856, and Mehrotra et al., p. 859.

Objectives. To examine the global prevalence of and factors associated with tobacco dependence among adolescents who are currently smoking.

Methods. We obtained 2012 to 2019 Global Youth Tobacco Survey data on 67 406 adolescents aged 12 to 16 years from 125 countries or territories (hereafter countries). Those with tobacco dependence were defined as current smokers who felt a strong desire to smoke again within 24 hours after smoking or who had ever smoked or felt like smoking first thing in the morning.

Results. The global prevalence of tobacco dependence among adolescents who were currently smoking was 38.4% (95% confidence interval [CI] = 34.0, 42.7). The prevalence was highest in high-income countries (49.8%; 95% CI = 47.0, 52.6) and lowest in lower-middle-income countries (31.2%; 95% CI = 26.9, 35.4). Secondhand smoke exposure, parental smoking, smoking among closest friends, tobacco advertisement exposure, and offers of free tobacco products were positively associated with tobacco dependence.

Conclusions. Nearly 40% of adolescents who are currently smoking have tobacco dependence worldwide.

Public Health Implications. Our findings emphasize the need to develop tobacco control interventions to prevent experimentation from progressing to regular smoking among adolescents who are currently smoking tobacco. (*Am J Public Health.* 2023;113(8):861–869. https://doi.org/10.2105/AJPH.2023.307283)

AJPH August 2023, Vol 113, No. 8

Tobacco use is one of the leading causes of preventable chronic noncommunicable diseases and premature death, killing an estimated 8.7 million people per year worldwide.[1] Globally, about 70% of adult smokers start smoking during their childhood or adolescence.[2] Adolescent smoking continues to be a severe problem, with the prevalence of current tobacco use among adolescents (13–15 years old) either increasing or remaining unchanged in more than half of 137 countries and territories from 1999 to 2019.[3] In addition, the current prevalence of any tobacco use (including either cigarettes or other tobacco products) on at least 1 day during the past 30 days globally among adolescents is estimated to be 17.9% among boys and 11.5% among girls.[3]

Nicotine in tobacco products is highly addictive, and adolescents are especially sensitive to nicotine addiction because their brains are not fully developed.[4] At present, most tobacco control strategies and measures targeting adolescents focus on prevention of initiation; however, as a result of tobacco dependence, most adolescents who have already smoked for some time usually have difficulty in quitting smoking.[5] According to the *International Classification of Diseases, 10th Revision* (*ICD-10*) and the latest edition of the *Diagnostic and Statistical Manual of Mental Disorders*, tobacco dependence is considered a mental health disorder[6,7] characterized by increased tolerance and withdrawal symptoms such as craving and anxiety.[7,8] Among adolescents, tobacco dependence can impair their brain development,[4] lead to emotional disorders and substance abuse,[9,10] and increase the risk of tobacco-related illness and death in adulthood.[11]

Tobacco dependence is common but often overlooked, especially among young people who are currently smoking tobacco.[7,12,13] Chronic and frequent use has previously been considered a prerequisite of tobacco dependence, but recent studies have shown that some adolescents develop symptoms of tobacco dependence after brief, intermittent use, even 1 or 2 cigarettes.[14] The reported prevalence of tobacco dependence at the national level among adolescents who use tobacco ranges from 22.0% in Lebanon to 87.0% in Cyprus[11,15–17] according to different diagnostic criteria and study populations. However, to our knowledge, there is no global prevalence estimate of tobacco dependence among adolescents who are currently smoking tobacco. It has been reported that the earlier one starts smoking, the less likely one can quit and the more likely the smoking habit continues to adulthood.[4,18]

Of note, environmental and social factors (e.g., parental smoking and peer smoking) are known to be associated with the development of adolescent tobacco dependence.[19] However, other factors associated with adolescent tobacco dependence are poorly understood. Therefore, monitoring the prevalence of tobacco dependence among adolescents who are currently smoking tobacco and its related factors is of great importance in preventing the transition from experimentation to regular smoking and in guiding cessation of smoking among adolescents who are currently smoking tobacco.

Using globally representative data from the Global Youth Tobacco Survey (GYTS), we aimed to assess the global prevalence in 125 countries and territories (hereafter countries) of tobacco dependence among adolescents aged 12 to 16 years who are currently smoking tobacco and to examine factors potentially associated with adolescent tobacco dependence.

METHODS

We obtained 2012 to 2019 GYTS data from 125 countries on tobacco dependence among adolescents aged 12 to 16 years who were currently smoking tobacco. The GYTS is a nationality representative and ongoing school-based surveillance survey focusing on tobacco use and associated factors among adolescents worldwide. Each participating country follows the same 2-stage sampling method: schools are randomly selected based on enrollment size in the first stage, and classes are randomly selected from the selected schools in the second stage. All included students voluntarily and anonymously complete a standardized questionnaire with the same set of core questions. The GYTS is organized jointly by the World Health Organization (WHO) and the US Centers for Disease Control and Prevention (further information on the GYTS is available at https://www.cdc.gov/tobacco/global/gtss/gtssdata/index.html). It should be noted that the related GYTS data in China were not publicly available, and thus we retrieved information on China from the 2014 Chinese Youth Tobacco Survey[20] (part of the GYTS).

After exclusion of participants with missing data on age (n = 2673), sex (n = 4516), and 2 measures of tobacco dependence (n = 1035); those aged 11 years or younger (n = 8102) or 17 years or older (n = 36 738); and those who were not currently smoking tobacco (n = 457 332), our data analysis included 67 406 adolescents aged 12 to 16 years who were currently smoking tobacco in 125 countries from 2012 to 2019.

Definitions of Tobacco Smoking and Dependence

Current tobacco smoking status was defined as smoking either cigarettes or other tobacco products on 1 or more days during the past 30 days on the basis of responses to the following 2 questions: "During the past 30 days, on how many days did you smoke cigarettes?" and "During the past 30 days, have you ever used any form of smoked tobacco products other than cigarettes (such as cigars, little cigar, pipe)?"

Consistent with the 2014 Chinese Youth Tobacco Survey report,[20] those with tobacco dependence were defined as current tobacco smokers who felt a strong desire to smoke again within 24 hours after smoking tobacco or who had ever smoked tobacco or felt like smoking tobacco first thing in the morning (sometimes or always). This definition was based on responses to 2 questions: "How soon after you smoke tobacco do you start to feel a strong desire to smoke again that is hard to ignore?" (response options were never, within 2 hours, more than 2 hours but less than 1 full day, and 1 day or more) and "Do you ever smoke tobacco or feel like smoking tobacco first thing in the morning?" (response options were no; yes, sometimes; and yes, always). Responses were coded as "yes" for tobacco dependence if current tobacco smokers reported a strong desire to smoke again after smoking tobacco within 24 hours or reported that they ever smoked tobacco or felt like smoking tobacco first thing in the morning; otherwise, responses were coded as "no."

Definitions of Potential Associated Factors

Secondhand smoke exposure was defined as exposure to secondhand smoke at any place on 1 or more days during the past 7 days according to responses to the following 3 questions: (1) "During the past 7 days, on how many days has anyone smoked in your presence inside your home?" (2) "During the past 7 days, on how many days has anyone smoked in your presence inside any enclosed public place?" and (3) "During the past 7 days, on how many days has anyone smoked in your presence at any outdoor public place?"

Parental smoking status was assessed with the question "Do your parents smoke tobacco?" (response options were both, father only, mother only, and neither). The smoking status of participants' closest friends was assessed with the question "Do any of your closest friends smoke tobacco?" (response options were none, some, most, and all).

Tobacco advertisement exposure was defined as exposure to 1 or more sources of tobacco advertisements based on responses to the following 3 questions: (1) "During the past 30 days, did you see any people using tobacco on TV, in movies, or in videos?" (2) "During the past 30 days, did you see any advertisements or promotions for tobacco products at points of sale?" and (3) "Do you have something with a tobacco product brand logo on it?" Participants who responded yes to the question "Has a person working for a tobacco company ever offered you a free tobacco product?" were classified as being offered free tobacco products. Information on the income level of each country was extracted from the World Bank classification Web site corresponding to the GYTS survey year.

Statistical Analysis

We calculated all prevalence or proportion estimates and 95% confidence intervals (CIs) in participating countries using original sampling weights with consideration of strata and primary sampling units owing to the complex sampling survey. Overall and subgroup estimates and 95% confidence intervals were calculated with rescaled weights in consideration of the sample size in each country. We used the χ^2 test to examine differences in prevalence or proportion estimates between subgroups (sex, age group, WHO region, and World Bank income category). A stepwise regression method was used to analyze all potential associated factors and to screen out meaningful factors. We used a multivariable logistic regression model to examine the association of tobacco dependence among adolescents who were currently smoking tobacco with identified factors (age, secondhand smoke exposure, parental smoking, smoking among closest friends, tobacco advertisement exposure, and offers of free tobacco products).

All identified factors were introduced simultaneously into the multivariable logistic regression model. Information on the code for each variable is shown in Table A (available as a supplement to the online version of this article at http://www.ajph.org). We used SAS version 9.4 (SAS Institute Inc, Cary, NC) in conducting our data analysis and considered 2-sided *P* values less than .05 as indicating statistical significance.

RESULTS

As noted, 67 406 adolescents aged 12 to 16 years from 125 countries who were currently smoking tobacco (70.1% boys) were included in our data analysis. Table B (available as a supplement to the online version of this article at http://www.ajph.org) presents data on the characteristics of the participants (who were from 20 [16.0%] WHO African region countries, 25 [20.0%] American region countries, 20 [16.0%] Eastern Mediterranean region countries, 32 [25.6%] European region countries, 7 [5.6%] Southeast Asian region countries, and 21 [16.8%] Western Pacific region countries).

About 27% (95% CI = 20.6, 32.5) of adolescents who were currently smoking tobacco reported that they had a strong desire to smoke again within 2 hours after smoking, and 13.1% (95% CI = 8.1, 18.1) reported that they had a strong desire in 2 to 24 hours. The proportions of adolescents who had a strong desire to smoke again after smoking were similar between male and female smokers and between those aged 12 to 14 years and those aged 15 to 16 years (Table 1). Time intervals of strong desire among adolescents who were currently smoking tobacco varied significantly across countries (Table C, available as a

TABLE 1— Time Intervals to Strong Desire to Smoke Again After Tobacco Smoking Among Adolescents Aged 12–16 Years Who Were Currently Smoking Tobacco, by Sex, Age Group, WHO Region, and World Bank Income Category: 2012–2019

Group	No. of Countries	<2 Hours			2–24 Hours			>24 Hours		
		Total	Boys	Girls	Total	Boys	Girls	Total	Boys	Girls
Total, % (95% CI)	125	26.5 (20.6, 32.5)	27.7 (19.7, 35.7)	23.3 (20.1, 26.5)	13.1 (8.1, 18.1)	14.2 (7.5, 20.9)	10.2 (7.5, 12.8)	12.2 (10.3, 14.0)	12.2 (9.7, 14.8)	12.0 (10.3, 13.7)
Age group, y, % (95% CI)										
12–14	125	27.2 (16.3, 38.1)	28.5 (14.0, 42.9)	23.6 (19.3, 27.8)	13.8 (4.8, 22.8)	15.5 (3.6, 27.4)	9.1 (5.2, 13.0)	10.8 (8.4, 13.2)	10.7 (7.5, 13.9)	11.0 (8.8, 13.3)
15–16	125	25.8 (22.9, 28.7)	26.8 (23.3, 30.3)	23.1 (18.8, 27.3)	12.4 (9.7, 15.0)	12.7 (9.2, 16.3)	11.3 (8.4, 14.3)	13.7 (11.2, 16.2)	14.0 (10.7, 17.3)	13.0 (10.4, 15.7)
P		.8	.82	.86	.75	.64	.36	.07	.12	.25
WHO region, % (95% CI)										
Africa	20	30.1 (25.5, 34.8)	29.4 (23.7, 35.0)	32.0 (23.2, 40.7)	11.2 (5.5, 16.9)	12.5 (4.8, 20.2)	8.1 (2.7, 13.4)	9.8 (7.3, 12.3)	10.7 (7.4, 14.1)	7.6 (3.8, 11.4)
Americas	25	21.3 (15.9, 26.8)	20.5 (14.8, 26.1)	22.3 (15.0, 29.6)	10.3 (5.0, 15.6)	9.0 (4.2, 13.7)	11.8 (5.0, 18.6)	13.6 (11.6, 15.6)	13.3 (10.5, 16.1)	14.0 (10.6, 17.4)
Eastern Mediterranean	20	24.0 (18.8, 29.1)	26.2 (20.2, 32.1)	15.2[a] (9.5, 20.9)	15.3 (7.4, 23.1)	17.9 (8.7, 27.1)	4.7[a] (1.9, 7.4)	15.9 (11.6, 20.2)	16.9 (11.4, 22.3)	12.0 (6.9, 17.1)
Europe	32	25.4 (23.2, 27.7)	25.6 (22.2, 28.9)	25.3 (21.9, 28.7)	13.1 (11.3, 15.0)	13.2 (10.7, 15.6)	13.1 (9.8, 16.3)	12.4 (10.1, 14.7)	11.3 (9.2, 13.5)	13.6 (10.2, 17.0)
Southeast Asia	7	30.5 (12.3, 48.7)	31.8 (12.3, 51.3)	15.9[a] (7.3, 24.5)	15.8 (0.6, 31.1)	16.5 (0.0, 33.1)	8.1[a] (2.5, 13.8)	11.2 (5.7, 16.7)	11.1 (5.2, 17.1)	12.2 (4.3, 20.0)
Western Pacific	21	22.6 (19.5, 25.7)	22.8 (19.2, 26.5)	21.9 (16.4, 27.4)	9.7 (7.7, 11.7)	9.8 (7.6, 11.9)	9.4 (5.1, 13.7)	10.5 (8.1, 12.9)	11.0 (8.2, 13.8)	8.8 (4.8, 12.8)
P		.59	.61	.018	.85	.76	.25	.29	.38	.22
World Bank income category, % (95% CI)										
Low	19	38.6 (15.9, 61.4)	40.4 (13.4, 67.4)	30.0 (18.9, 41.2)	18.0 (0.0, 38.6)	21.1 (0.0, 45.6)	2.9[a] (0.0, 6.7)	9.2 (3.0, 15.5)	9.7 (2.1, 17.2)	7.2 (1.9, 12.4)
Lower middle	36	19.9 (17.0, 22.7)	20.2 (16.8, 23.7)	18.0 (13.5, 22.6)	10.3 (7.2, 13.5)	10.8 (7.1, 14.6)	8.1 (4.7, 11.5)	12.4 (9.8, 15.1)	13.4 (10.2, 16.7)	7.7[a] (5.3, 10.1)
Upper middle	39	25.1 (21.5, 28.7)	27.1 (23.5, 30.7)	22.0 (15.7, 28.2)	12.3 (8.4, 16.2)	12.6 (8.7, 16.4)	12.0 (6.2, 17.7)	13.4 (11.6, 15.3)	12.5 (10.4, 14.6)	14.8 (11.5, 18.1)
High	31	28.2 (25.6, 30.8)	28.6 (24.5, 32.7)	27.6 (24.0, 31.3)	14.7 (12.7, 16.6)	14.9 (12.3, 17.5)	14.4 (10.8, 17.9)	14.0 (11.7, 16.3)	13.0 (10.7, 15.3)	15.2 (11.6, 18.8)
P		.036	.06	.07	.63	.47	.022	.43	.66	.004

Note. CI = confidence interval; WHO = World Health Organization.

[a]Statistically significant difference between sexes.

supplement to the online version of this article at http://www.ajph.org) and by WHO region and World Bank income category (Table 1).

About 32% (95% CI = 27.6, 35.9) of adolescents who were currently smoking tobacco reported that they sometimes smoked tobacco or felt like smoking tobacco first thing in the morning, and 8.0% (95% CI = 6.2, 9.8) reported that they always did. The proportions of adolescents who reported that they sometimes or always smoked tobacco or felt like smoking tobacco first thing in the morning were higher among those aged 15 to 16 years than among those aged 12 to 14 years (Table 2). These proportions also varied significantly across countries (Table D, available as a supplement to the online version of this article at http://www.ajph.org) and by WHO region and World Bank income category (Table 2).

As shown in Table E (available as a supplement to the online version of this article at http://www.ajph.org), 27.8% (95% CI = 24.9, 30.6) of adolescents who were currently smoking cigarettes reported that they had smoked 2 to 5 cigarettes per day in the past 30 days, and 13.3% (95% CI = 11.5, 15.1) reported that they had smoked 6 or more cigarettes per day. The intensity of cigarette smoking in the past 30 days varied significantly by WHO region and World Bank income category.

The overall global prevalence of tobacco dependence (defined by the strong desire to smoke again within 24 hours after smoking or sometimes or always smoking tobacco or feeling like smoking tobacco first thing in the morning) among adolescents who were currently smoking tobacco was 38.4% (95% CI = 34.0, 42.7). The prevalence was higher among male smokers (40.6%; 95% CI = 34.8, 46.3) than female smokers (33.1%; 95% CI = 29.4, 36.8) and somewhat higher among those aged 15 to 16 years (40.0%; 95% CI = 37.1, 43.0) than among those aged 12 to 14 years (37.0%; 95% CI = 29.7, 44.4).

The prevalence of tobacco dependence was highest in the Southeast Asian region (46.4%; 95% CI = 34.0, 58.7) and lowest in the Eastern Mediterranean region (29.1%; 95%

AJPH August 2023, Vol 113, No. 8

TABLE 2— Percentages of Adolescents Aged 12–16 Years Who Were Currently Smoking Tobacco and Ever Smoked Tobacco or Felt Like Smoking Tobacco First Thing in the Morning, by Sex, Age Group, WHO Region, and World Bank Income Category: 2012–2019

Group	No. of Countries	Sometimes			Always		
		Total	Boys	Girls	Total	Boys	Girls
Total, % (95% CI)	125	31.8 (27.6, 35.9)	32.3 (26.5, 38.1)	30.5 (27.0, 34.0)	8.0 (6.2, 9.8)	8.2 (5.9, 10.6)	7.5 (5.7, 9.3)
Age group, y, % (95% CI)							
12–14	125	31.5 (24.5, 38.5)	32.4 (22.7, 42.0)	29.5 (24.3, 34.7)	5.6 (4.0, 7.1)	5.5 (3.5, 7.4)	5.8 (3.5, 8.1)
15–16	125	32.1 (28.4, 35.7)	32.2 (27.5, 36.9)	31.7 (27.5, 35.9)	10.9 (7.9, 13.9)	11.4 (7.5, 15.3)	9.6 (7.0, 12.3)
P		.9	.97	.53	< .001	< .001	.029
WHO region, % (95% CI)							
Africa	20	28.3 (24.2, 32.4)	29.2 (23.6, 34.8)	26.4 (17.9, 34.8)	12.1 (8.5, 15.8)	10.7 (6.4, 15.0)	15.3 (8.1, 22.6)
Americas	25	33.1 (27.8, 38.4)	28.2 (22.0, 34.4)	39.0[a] (31.6, 46.3)	4.9 (3.1, 6.7)	5.8 (3.2, 8.4)	3.9 (2.1, 5.7)
Eastern Mediterranean	20	36.6 (25.6, 47.5)	40.6 (27.8, 53.4)	20.6[a] (13.4, 27.8)	8.5 (5.5, 11.4)	9.6 (6.0, 13.1)	4.1[a] (1.6, 6.7)
Europe	32	31.5 (28.6, 34.4)	27.5 (24.0, 31.0)	35.9[a] (31.8, 40.1)	12.1 (10.3, 13.9)	12.9 (10.2, 15.5)	11.2 (8.5, 13.9)
Southeast Asia	7	32.8 (20.6, 44.9)	35.1 (20.8, 49.3)	18.2[a] (6.7, 29.7)	6.4 (1.4, 11.5)	6.9 (1.2, 12.7)	3.2 (0.0, 7.4)
Western Pacific	21	24.5 (21.3, 27.8)	23.8 (20.1, 27.4)	26.8 (20.2, 33.4)	5.1 (3.2, 7.0)	5.2 (3.2, 7.2)	4.8 (1.8, 7.8)
P		.59	.24	< .001	.009	.21	< .001
World Bank income category, % (95% CI)							
Low	19	31.9 (17.0, 46.7)	37.5 (17.8, 57.2)	15.6[a] (7.4, 23.8)	9.1 (2.7, 15.4)	9.2 (0.8, 17.6)	8.6 (3.3, 13.9)
Lower middle	36	29.0 (24.2, 33.7)	29.8 (24.3, 35.4)	25.0 (20.3, 29.7)	6.0 (4.2, 7.8)	5.6 (3.7, 7.4)	8.0 (3.8, 12.2)
Upper middle	39	33.6 (29.5, 37.7)	31.0 (26.1, 36.0)	37.5 (31.0, 44.1)	8.5 (6.0, 11.0)	10.8 (7.4, 14.1)	5.0[a] (2.8, 7.3)
High	31	36.4 (33.6, 39.3)	32.7 (29.0, 36.4)	40.8[a] (36.3, 45.2)	11.1 (9.2, 13.0)	11.7 (8.9, 14.4)	10.5 (7.8, 13.2)
P		.69	.7	< .001	.28	.22	.17

Note. CI = confidence interval; WHO = World Health Organization.

[a]Statistically significant difference between sexes.

CI = 20.7, 37.4) and highest in high-income countries (49.8%; 95% CI = 47.0, 52.6) and lowest in lower-middle-income countries (31.2%; 95% CI = 26.9, 35.4; Table 3). The prevalence ranged from 0.0% in Turkmenistan to 66.4% in Finland and varied significantly by sex and age group across all the included countries (Figure A, Figure B, and Table F, available as supplements to the online version of this article at http://www.ajph.org).

Secondhand smoke exposure (vs no exposure; odds ratio [OR] = 2.12; 95% CI = 1.61, 2.80), both parents smoking (vs neither; OR = 1.63; 95% CI = 1.32, 2.01), smoking among closest friends (vs none; some: OR = 1.85; 95% CI = 1.46, 2.35; most: OR = 3.86; 95% CI = 3.03, 4.92; all: OR = 6.05; 95% CI = 4.12, 8.88), exposure to tobacco advertisements (vs no exposure; OR = 1.29; 95% CI = 1.04, 1.60), and offers of free tobacco products (vs no offers; OR = 1.49; 95% CI = 1.13, 1.98) were all positively associated with tobacco dependence among adolescents who were currently smoking tobacco (Table 4). Subgroup analyses by age group showed similar results (Table G, available as a supplement to the online version of this article at http://www.ajph.org).

DISCUSSION

We found that nearly 40% of adolescents who were currently smoking tobacco had a strong desire to smoke again within 24 hours after smoking. Craving is the primary manifestation of tobacco dependence as defined by the *ICD-10*.[6] Among adolescents, craving is the most common and severe withdrawal symptom.[21–23] Craving is significantly associated with tobacco consumption among adolescents[23] and can predict dependence severity and likelihood of relapse.[23–25]

In addition, nearly 40% of adolescents who were currently smoking tobacco reported ever smoking or feeling like smoking first thing in the morning. Because of the short half-life of nicotine (about 2 hours), the majority of smokers wake up in a nicotine-deprived state in the morning,[26] and thus tobacco-dependent smokers will have their first cigarette or other tobacco product as soon as they wake up.[27] Time to first cigarette has been considered the best single-item index of nicotine dependence.[28,29] Earlier time to first cigarette is associated with greater severity of tobacco dependence and a greater likelihood of failure to quit smoking.[29] Strong desire and time to first cigarette have been identified as

TABLE 3— Prevalence of Tobacco Dependence Among Adolescents Aged 12–16 Years Who Were Currently Smoking Tobacco, by Sex, Age Group, WHO Region, and World Bank Income Category: 2012–2019

Group	No. of Countries	Total	Boys	Girls	12–14 Years	15–16 Years
Total, % (95% CI)	125	38.4 (34.0, 42.7)	40.6 (34.8, 46.3)	33.1[a] (29.4, 36.8)	37.0 (29.7, 44.4)	40.0 (37.1, 43.0)
WHO region, % (95% CI)						
Africa	20	35.6 (31.3, 40.0)	36.6 (31.2, 42.0)	33.6 (25.8, 41.4)	30.6 (25.6, 35.6)	41.5[b] (34.1, 48.8)
Americas	25	38.8 (32.6, 45.1)	35.7 (29.5, 42.0)	42.4 (34.4, 50.4)	40.5 (32.9, 48.2)	37.3 (31.0, 43.7)
Eastern Mediterranean	20	29.1 (20.7, 37.4)	33.6 (22.9, 44.3)	14.4[a] (10.2, 18.5)	22.8 (14.5, 31.0)	37.1[b] (28.4, 45.8)
Europe	32	42.6 (39.7, 45.5)	40.5 (37.3, 43.6)	45.2[a] (40.9, 49.6)	37.1 (33.0, 41.3)	47.8[b] (44.3, 51.3)
Southeast Asia	7	46.4 (34.0, 58.7)	50.7 (37.4, 64.1)	19.9[a] (11.2, 28.6)	48.4 (31.2, 65.7)	42.0 (35.3, 48.8)
Western Pacific	21	31.9 (28.2, 35.6)	33.5 (29.2, 37.9)	27.7 (22.2, 33.3)	30.8 (25.8, 35.7)	33.0 (28.1, 37.9)
P		.006	.005	< .001	< .001	.12
World Bank income category, % (95% CI)						
Low	19	43.9 (29.5, 58.3)	51.3 (34.5, 68.2)	22.5[a] (15.5, 29.6)	49.6 (29.9, 69.2)	33.5 (25.6, 41.4)
Lower middle	36	31.2 (26.9, 35.4)	33.3 (28.1, 38.5)	23.5[a] (18.7, 28.3)	25.5 (21.3, 29.8)	38.4[b] (33.5, 43.3)
Upper middle	39	39.9 (35.4, 44.4)	40.3 (35.6, 44.9)	39.2 (32.3, 46.1)	38.0 (32.5, 43.5)	41.6 (36.4, 46.8)
High	31	49.8 (47.0, 52.6)	47.6 (43.8, 51.5)	52.5 (48.2, 56.7)	47.7 (43.5, 51.9)	51.7 (48.1, 55.3)
P		.01	.008	< .001	< .001	.005

Note. CI = confidence interval; WHO = World Health Organization.

[a]Statistically significant difference between sexes.
[b]Statistically significant difference between age groups.

TABLE 4— Potential Factors Associated With Tobacco Dependence Among Adolescents Aged 12–16 Years Who Were Currently Smoking Tobacco on the Basis of the Latest Available Data: 2012–2019

Variable	Prevalence, %	OR (95% CI)
Age group, y		
12–14	37.0	1 (Ref)
15–16	40.0	1.40 (1.19, 1.65)
Secondhand smoke exposure		
No	14.0	1 (Ref)
Yes	43.3	2.12 (1.61, 2.80)
Parental smoking		
Neither	32.2	1 (Ref)
Father only	42.3	1.08 (0.89, 1.31)
Mother only	49.3	1.36 (0.97, 1.93)
Both	50.2	1.63 (1.32, 2.01)
Smoking among closest friends		
None	21.2	1 (Ref)
Some	38.4	1.85 (1.46, 2.35)
Most	56.0	3.86 (3.03, 4.92)
All	65.6	6.05 (4.12, 8.88)
Tobacco advertisement exposure		
No	29.2	1 (Ref)
Yes	40.5	1.29 (1.04, 1.60)
Offers of free tobacco products		
No	36.7	1 (Ref)
Yes	45.5	1.49 (1.13, 1.98)

Note. CI = confidence interval; OR = odds ratio. All variables listed in the table were introduced into multivariable logistic regression models.

valid and reliable indicators of tobacco dependence among adolescents who are currently smoking tobacco.[30,31]

According to the 2 indicators just described, the global prevalence of tobacco dependence was quite high (approximately 40%) among adolescents who were currently smoking tobacco. To our knowledge, our study is the first to report on the global prevalence of tobacco dependence among adolescents who are currently smoking tobacco based on the most recent data. At the national level, the reported prevalence of tobacco dependence among adolescents ranges from 22.0% in Lebanon to 87.0% in Cyprus.[11,15–17] However, because of differences in the basic characteristics of participants and definitions of tobacco dependence, direct comparability between countries is poor.

In our study, based on comparable data in 125 countries, the prevalence of tobacco dependence among adolescents who were currently smoking tobacco varied greatly across countries, ranging from 0.0% in Turkmenistan to 66.4% in Finland, and the prevalence was highest in the Southeast Asian region and lowest in the Eastern Mediterranean region. Turkmenistan has made a significant contribution to the fight against smoking and has the lowest prevalence in the world, which should be of note to other countries globally.[32] Possible explanations for differences in the prevalence of tobacco dependence across WHO regions include diversity in the tobacco products primarily used,[33,34] genetic background,[35] and degree of acculturation.[19]

In addition, we found that the prevalence of tobacco dependence was highest in high-income countries and lowest in lower-middle-income countries. This finding might be explained by the "reinforcement hypothesis," according to which the prevalence of tobacco use may decline in areas where tobacco control policies are strict and the remaining smokers are mainly highly dependent ones.[36–39] Also, there is well-documented evidence of the effectiveness of tobacco control policies (e.g., tobacco tax increases) in reducing tobacco consumption, especially among adolescents and people with low incomes.[40] However, high levels of economic development in high-income countries might make tobacco more affordable for youths.[40]

Our findings underscore the necessity of tailor-made tobacco control strategies and measures considering the prevalence of tobacco dependence among adolescents who are currently smoking tobacco in different countries and World Bank regions. Moreover, it is essential to establish unified diagnostic criteria of tobacco dependence among adolescents who are currently smoking tobacco to allow early identification and timely treatment, especially in countries with a high prevalence of tobacco dependence.

In addition, we found a higher prevalence of tobacco dependence among older smokers than among younger ones, which might be explained by the accessibility of tobacco products.[41] Consistent with previous studies,[16,42] we also found that parental smoking, smoking among closest friends, tobacco advertisement exposure, and offers of free tobacco products were all positively associated with tobacco dependence among adolescents who were currently smoking tobacco. These findings can be explained by the social learning theory of substance use; that is, the progression from experimentation to dependence among adolescents who are currently smoking tobacco proceeds through imitation and social reinforcement.[41]

Notably, adolescents exposed to secondhand smoke were more likely to develop tobacco dependence. Secondhand smoke exposure, as well as smoking among closest friends, exerts social pressure on adolescents who may not smoke to adapt to their surroundings,[43] increases sensitivity to nicotine, and promotes desire.[44] Strict tobacco control strategies and measures (e.g., banning smoking in public places and regulating tobacco marketing) should be implemented to promote smoking cessation among adolescents who are currently smoking tobacco.

Strengths and Limitations

One strength of our study is that we used globally representative data including 67 406 adolescents from 125 countries who were currently smoking tobacco to evaluate the global prevalence of tobacco dependence. In addition, all countries used the same standardized questionnaire for data collection, making prevalence estimates between different countries directly comparable.

However, there are several limitations. First, data on tobacco dependence and associated factors were self-reported, and such reports may be prone to recall bias. Second, questions related to tobacco dependence did not involve smokeless tobacco, which may have led to an underestimation of tobacco dependence. Third, the definition of tobacco dependence was not based on WHO formal criteria because the GYTS did not provide related data. In addition, our study involved only 2 measures of tobacco dependence (strong desire and time to first cigarette); other measures (e.g., number of all tobacco products smoked per day) that could help to identify tobacco dependence were not included, and thus our data might not fully reflect the symptoms of tobacco dependence. Fourth, because of the cross-sectional design of the GYTS, it is impossible to assess the causal relationship between associated factors and tobacco dependence. Fifth, several factors (e.g., family income, residence, initiation age of smoking tobacco) that might be associated with adolescent tobacco dependence were not assessed because data were not available.

Conclusions

We found that nearly 40% of adolescents who were currently smoking tobacco reported tobacco dependence. On one hand, it is necessary to implement preventive strategies and measures for tobacco use among adolescents, preventing the transition from experimentation to regular smoking. On the other hand, health education programs on adolescent tobacco dependence are essential to identify tobacco dependence early and guide smoking cessation among adolescents who are currently smoking tobacco. In addition, trends in the prevalence of tobacco dependence among adolescents who are currently smoking tobacco should be assessed in the future to help policymakers make decisions. AJPH

ABOUT THE AUTHORS

Hui Yang, Chuanwei Ma, and Bo Xi are with the Department of Epidemiology, School of Public Health/Qilu Hospital, Cheeloo College of Medicine, Shandong University, Jinan, China. Min Zhao is with the Department of Nutrition and Food Hygiene, School of Public Health, Cheeloo College of Medicine, Shandong University.

CORRESPONDENCE

Correspondence should be sent to Bo Xi, MD, Department of Epidemiology, School of Public Health/Qilu Hospital, Cheeloo College of Medicine, Shandong University, 44 Wen Huaxi Rd, Jinan, 250012, China. (e-mail: xibo2007@126.com). Reprints can be ordered at http://www.ajph.org by clicking the "Reprints" link.

PUBLICATION INFORMATION

Full Citation: Yang H, Ma C, Zhao M, Xi B. Prevalence of and factors associated with tobacco dependence among adolescents aged 12–16 years who were currently smoking tobacco in 125 countries or territories, 2012–2019. *Am J Public Health*. 2023;113(8): 861–869.

Acceptance Date: March 9, 2023.

DOI: https://doi.org/10.2105/AJPH.2023.307283

CONTRIBUTORS

H. Yang conducted the statistical analysis and drafted the first version of the article. C. Ma, M. Zhao, and B. Xi critically revised the article. M. Zhao and B. Xi contributed to interpretation of findings. B. Xi designed the study and was the principal investigator.

ACKNOWLEDGMENTS

This study was supported by the Youth Team of Humanistic and Social Science of Shandong University (grant 20820IFYT1902).

We thank the World Health Organization (WHO) and the United States Centers for Disease Control and Prevention (CDC) for sharing the Global Youth Tobacco Survey data.

Note. The conclusions are those of the authors and do not represent the official position of WHO or the CDC.

CONFLICTS OF INTEREST

The authors declare no competing interests.

HUMAN PARTICIPANT PROTECTION

The Global Youth Tobacco Survey data sets are publicly available and do not include any individual identification data. All surveys have been reviewed by the corresponding national ethics committees, and all participants provided informed consent.

REFERENCES

1. GBD 2019 Risk Factors Collaborators. Global burden of 87 risk factors in 204 countries and territories, 1990–2019: a systematic analysis for the Global Burden of Disease Study 2019. *Lancet.* 2020;396(10258):1223–1249. https://doi.org/10.1016/S0140-6736(20)30752-2
2. Reitsma MB, Flor LS, Mullany EC, Gupta V, Hay SI, Gakidou E. Spatial, temporal, and demographic patterns in prevalence of smoking tobacco use and initiation among young people in 204 countries and territories, 1990–2019. *Lancet Public Health.* 2021;6(7):e472–e481. https://doi.org/10.1016/S2468-2667(21)00102-X
3. Ma C, Xi B, Li Z, et al. Prevalence and trends in tobacco use among adolescents aged 13–15 years in 143 countries, 1999–2018: findings from the Global Youth Tobacco Surveys. *Lancet Child Adolesc Health.* 2021;5(4):245–255. https://doi.org/10.1016/S2352-4642(20)30390-4
4. US Department of Health and Human Services. *Preventing Tobacco Use Among Youth and Young Adults: A Report of the Surgeon General.* Atlanta, GA: Centers for Disease Control and Prevention; 2012.
5. Prokhorov AV, Hudmon KS, Stancic N. Adolescent smoking: epidemiology and approaches for achieving cessation. *Paediatr Drugs.* 2003;5(1):1–10. https://doi.org/10.2165/00128072-200305010-00001
6. World Health Organization. International Statistical Classification of Diseases and Related Health Problems, 10th Revision. Available at: https://icd.who.int/browse10/2019/en#. Accessed July 22, 2022.
7. American Psychiatric Association. *Diagnostic and statistical manual of mental disorders.* 5th ed. Washington, DC: American Psychiatric Publishing; 2013.
8. Hughes JR, Hatsukami D. Signs and symptoms of tobacco withdrawal. *Arch Gen Psychiatry.* 1986;43(3):289–294. https://doi.org/10.1001/archpsyc.1986.01800030107013
9. Dudas RB, Hans K, Barabas K. Anxiety, depression and smoking in schoolchildren—implications for smoking prevention. *J R Soc Promot Health.* 2005;125(2):87–92. https://doi.org/10.1177/146642400512500213
10. McCabe SE, West BT, McCabe VV. Associations between early onset of e-cigarette use and cigarette smoking and other substance use among US adolescents: a national study. *Nicotine Tob Res.* 2018;20(8):923–930. https://doi.org/10.1093/ntr/ntx231
11. Gomez Y, Creamer M, Trivers KF, et al. Patterns of tobacco use and nicotine dependence among youth, United States, 2017–2018. *Prev Med.* 2020;141:106284. https://doi.org/10.1016/j.ypmed.2020.106284
12. Xiao D, Wang C. Tobacco dependence should be recognised as a lethal non-communicable disease. *BMJ.* 2019;365:l2204. https://doi.org/10.1136/bmj.l2204
13. Doubeni CA, Reed G, Difranza JR. Early course of nicotine dependence in adolescent smokers. *Pediatrics.* 2010;125(6):1127–1133. https://doi.org/10.1542/peds.2009-0238
14. O'Loughlin J, DiFranza J, Tyndale RF, et al. Nicotine-dependence symptoms are associated with smoking frequency in adolescents. *Am J Prev Med.* 2003;25(3):219–225. https://doi.org/10.1016/S0749-3797(03)00198-3
15. Apelberg BJ, Corey CG, Hoffman AC, et al. Symptoms of tobacco dependence among middle and high school tobacco users: results from the 2012 National Youth Tobacco Survey. *Am J Prev Med.* 2014;47(suppl 1):S4–S14. https://doi.org/10.1016/j.amepre.2014.04.013
16. Christophi CA, Pampaka D, Paisi M, Ioannou S, DiFranza JR. Levels of physical dependence on tobacco among adolescent smokers in Cyprus. *Addict Behav.* 2016;60:148–153. https://doi.org/10.1016/j.addbeh.2016.04.004
17. Ebrahimi Kalan M, Behaleh R, DiFranza JR, et al. Natural course of nicotine dependence among adolescent waterpipe and cigarette smokers. *J Adolesc Health.* 2020;67(6):859–867. https://doi.org/10.1016/j.jadohealth.2020.04.030
18. Chassin L, Presson CC, Sherman SJ, Edwards DA. The natural history of cigarette smoking: predicting young-adult smoking outcomes from adolescent smoking patterns. *Health Psychol.* 1990;9(6):701–716. https://doi.org/10.1037/0278-6133.9.6.701
19. Mayhew KP, Flay BR, Mott JA. Stages in the development of adolescent smoking. *Drug Alcohol Depend.* 2000;59(suppl 1):S61–S81. https://doi.org/10.1016/S0376-8716(99)00165-9
20. Liang X, Xiao L, Jiang Y, et al. *Chinese Youth Tobacco Survey Report 2014.* Beijing, China: People's Medical Publishing House; 2014.
21. McNeill AD, West RJ, Jarvis M, Jackson P, Bryant A. Cigarette withdrawal symptoms in adolescent smokers. *Psychopharmacology (Berl).* 1986;90(4):533–536. https://doi.org/10.1007/BF00174074
22. Centers for Disease Control and Prevention. Reasons for tobacco use and symptoms of nicotine withdrawal among adolescent and young adult tobacco users—United States, 1993. *MMWR Morb Mortal Wkly Rep.* 1994;43(41):745–750.
23. Rojas NL, Killen JD, Haydel KF, Robinson TN. Nicotine dependence among adolescent smokers. *Arch Pediatr Adolesc Med.* 1998;152(2):151–156. https://doi.org/10.1001/archpedi.152.2.151
24. Killen JD, Fortmann SP, Kraemer HC, Varady A, Newman B. Who will relapse? Symptoms of nicotine dependence predict long-term relapse after smoking cessation. *J Consult Clin Psychol.* 1992;60(5):797–801. https://doi.org/10.1037/0022-006X.60.5.797
25. Siqueira LM, Rolnitzky LM, Rickert VI. Smoking cessation in adolescents: the role of nicotine dependence, stress, and coping methods. *Arch Pediatr Adolesc Med.* 2001;155(4):489–495. https://doi.org/10.1001/archpedi.155.4.489
26. Lynn T. Tobacco dependence, restraint and time to the first cigarette of the day. *Addict Behav.* 1981;6(4):307–312. https://doi.org/10.1016/0306-4603(81)90044-7
27. Heatherton TF, Kozlowski LT, Frecker RC, Fagerström KO. The Fagerström Test for Nicotine Dependence: a revision of the Fagerström Tolerance Questionnaire. *Br J Addict.* 1991;86(9):1119–1127. https://doi.org/10.1111/j.1360-0443.1991.tb01879.x
28. Baker TB, Piper ME, McCarthy DE, et al. Time to first cigarette in the morning as an index of ability to quit smoking: implications for nicotine dependence. *Nicotine Tob Res.* 2007;9(suppl 4):S555–S570. https://doi.org/10.1080/14622200701673480
29. Branstetter SA, Muscat JE, Mercincavage M. Time to first cigarette: a potential clinical screening tool for nicotine dependence. *J Addict Med.* 2020;14(5):409–414. https://doi.org/10.1097/ADM.0000000000000610
30. O'Loughlin J, Tarasuk J, Difranza J, Paradis G. Reliability of selected measures of nicotine dependence among adolescents. *Ann Epidemiol.* 2002;12(5):353–362. https://doi.org/10.1016/S1047-2797(01)00312-X
31. Nonnemaker J, Mowery P, Hersey J, et al. Measurement properties of a nicotine dependence scale for adolescents. *Nicotine Tob Res.* 2004;6(2):295–301. https://doi.org/10.1080/14622200410001676413
32. Bagcchi S. Turkmenistan bans tobacco sales. *Lancet Respir Med.* 2016;4(3):180. https://doi.org/10.1016/S2213-2600(16)00047-3
33. Sinha DN, Gupta PC, Kumar A, et al. The poorest of poor suffer the greatest burden from smokeless tobacco use: a study from 140 countries. *Nicotine Tob Res.* 2018;20(12):1529–1532. https://doi.org/10.1093/ntr/ntx276
34. Jawad M, Lee JT, Millett C. Waterpipe tobacco smoking prevalence and correlates in 25 Eastern Mediterranean and Eastern European countries: cross-sectional analysis of the Global Youth Tobacco Survey. *Nicotine Tob Res.* 2016;18(4):395–402. https://doi.org/10.1093/ntr/ntv101
35. Sullivan PF, Kendler KS. The genetic epidemiology of smoking. *Nicotine Tob Res.* 1999;1(suppl 2):S51–S57. https://doi.org/10.1080/14622299050011811
36. Allen JA, Gritz ER, Xiao H, et al. Impact of tobacco control policy on quitting and nicotine dependence among women in five European countries. *Tob Control.* 2014;23(2):173–177. https://doi.org/10.1136/tobaccocontrol-2011-050391
37. Malone RE, Warner KE. Tobacco control at twenty: reflecting on the past, considering the present and developing the new conversations for the future. *Tob Control.* 2012;21(2):74–76. https://doi.org/10.1136/tobaccocontrol-2012-050447
38. Docherty G, McNeill A, Gartner C, Szatkowski L. Did hardening occur among smokers in England from 2000 to 2010? *Addiction.* 2014;109(1):147–154. https://doi.org/10.1111/add.12359
39. Warner KE, Burns DM. Hardening and the hard-core smoker: concepts, evidence, and implications. *Nicotine Tob Res.* 2003;5(1):37–48. https://doi.org/10.1080/1462220021000060428
40. Drope JSN, Cahn Z, Drope J, Hamill S, Islami F. The tobacco atlas. Available at: https://tobaccoatlas.org. Accessed January 3, 2023.
41. Petraitis J, Flay BR, Miller TQ. Reviewing theories of adolescent substance use: organizing pieces in the puzzle. *Psychol Bull.* 1995;117(1):67–86. https://doi.org/10.1037/0033-2909.117.1.67
42. Flay BR, Hu FB, Siddiqui O, et al. Differential influence of parental smoking and friends' smoking on adolescent initiation and escalation of smoking. *J Health Soc Behav.* 1994;35(3):248–265. https://doi.org/10.2307/2137279
43. McGrath JJ, Racicot S, Okoli CTC, Hammond SK, O'Loughlin J. Airborne nicotine, secondhand smoke, and precursors to adolescent smoking. *Pediatrics.* 2018;141(suppl 1):S63–S74. https://doi.org/10.1542/peds.2017-1026J
44. Othman M, Farid NDN, Aghamohammadi N, Danaee M. Determinants of smokeless tobacco use and prevalence among Sudanese adolescents. *Arch Public Health.* 2021;79(1):176. https://doi.org/10.1186/s13690-021-00699-w

The Pent-Up Demand for Breastfeeding Among US Women: Trends After COVID-19 Shelter-in-Place

Rita Hamad, MD, PhD, Daniel F. Collin, MPH, Alison Gemmill, PhD, MPH, Kaitlyn Jackson, MPH, and Deborah Karasek, PhD, MPH

AJPH August 2023, Vol 113, No. 8

Objectives. To estimate changes in national breastfeeding trends immediately before and after COVID-19–related workplace closures in early 2020.

Methods. The implementation of shelter-in-place policies in early 2020, when 90% of people in the United States were urged to remain at home, represents a unique natural experiment to assess the pent-up demand for breastfeeding among US women that may be stymied by the lack of a national paid leave policy. We used the 2017–2020 Pregnancy Risk Assessment Monitoring System (n = 118 139) to estimate changes in breastfeeding practices for births occurring before and after shelter-in-place policies were implemented in the United States. We did this in the overall sample and by racial/ethnic and income subgroups.

Results. There was no change in breastfeeding initiation and a 17.5% increase in breastfeeding duration after shelter-in-place, with lingering effects through late 2020. High-income and White women demonstrated the largest gains.

Conclusions. The United States ranks worse than similar countries when it comes to breastfeeding initiation and duration. This study suggests that this is partly attributable to inadequate access to postpartum paid leave. This study also demonstrates inequities introduced by patterns of remote work during the pandemic. (*Am J Public Health*. 2023;113(8):870–873. https://doi.org/10.2105/AJPH.2023.307313)

The importance of breastfeeding for health has been increasingly recognized, with evidence suggesting benefits for both infants and parents.[1] The United States ranks near the bottom compared with similar countries when it comes to the prevalence and duration of breastfeeding. In the most recent harmonized data from the Organization for Economic Cooperation and Development in 2005, 31.5% of US babies were exclusively breastfed at 3 months, compared with 47.4% in other countries.[2] While US breastfeeding rates have increased in recent years, with 45% of babies exclusively breastfed at 3 months in 2019, they still fall short of peer countries and fail to meet national guidelines: the American Academy of Pediatrics recommends exclusive breastfeeding for 6 months.[3,4]

Moreover, substantial disparities exist, with lower breastfeeding rates among Black and low-income women.[5] While some face medical and personal challenges, and cultural differences are often blamed, structural barriers are a main reason for lagging breastfeeding rates, including lack of paid parental leave.[6,7] The United States is the only high-income country (and one of only a handful of countries worldwide) without a national paid family leave (PFL) policy for new mothers, and it is one of a few that does not provide paid leave to new fathers. As a consequence, only 25% of US private industry workers in 2022 had access to PFL through their employer.[8] In some cases, state policies support PFL: 9 states and Washington, DC, have implemented PFL policies, and 4 more have passed laws that are yet to be implemented. People of color and low-wage workers are the least likely to have access to PFL, forcing many to return to work to support their families.[9]

The degree to which breastfeeding rates would increase if working parents had access to leave is unknown. Births occurring immediately before COVID-19–related workplace closures, therefore, represent a unique natural experiment. During April 2020 shelter-in-place policies, 90% of people in the United States were urged to remain at home.[10] We examined national trends during this period of reduced in-person work to estimate the pent-up demand for breastfeeding.

METHODS

We used data from the 2017–2020 waves of the Pregnancy Risk Assessment Monitoring System (PRAMS), which links survey and birth certificate data from a national sample of postpartum people in the United States. We restricted the sample to PRAMS sites that collected data on the variables of interest during the study period (n = 118 139; see sample selection flowchart in Appendix Figure A, available as a supplement to the online version of this article at http://ajph.org). The 2 main outcomes were (1) whether the child was ever breastfed and (2) breastfeeding length (in weeks), excluding those who never breastfed.

We first examined characteristics for the sample overall and by time period. We next graphed trends by delivery month for the overall sample and by racial/ethnic and income subgroups. Next, we estimated the prevalence of breastfeeding and mean breastfeeding length in the overall sample and by subgroup for births occurring during 2 periods: (1) before shelter-in-place and (2) at the peak of shelter-in-place. For breastfeeding initiation, shelter-in-place policies would have most strongly affected births taking place in April and May 2020, because shelter-in-place orders across the country were mostly implemented in April 2020. We therefore considered births during April and May the "peak" against which we calculated absolute and relative differences. For breastfeeding duration, the mean was about 12 weeks, so that babies in April and May 2020 would have been born in January and February 2020. We therefore considered births during January and February to be the "peak" against which we calculated absolute and relative differences for this outcome. We used PRAMS survey weights to carry out the analysis.

Finally, we carried out a more sophisticated analysis to examine whether these trends were statistically significantly different from prepandemic trends. Specifically, we employed a Bayesian structural time-series approach (implemented using the CausalImpact package in R [R Foundation for Statistical Computing, Vienna, Austria]), similar to traditional interrupted time-series approaches that account for trends or other temporal patterns in the data.[11] This also allowed us to examine the longer-term trends after the peak period and whether any discontinuities were sustained throughout 2020. This method has been previously used to examine the effect of COVID-19 containment policies,[12] and details are provided in the "Supplemental Methods" in the Appendix.

RESULTS

Nearly two thirds (58.2%) of the sample were White, with 15.8% Black, 16.5% Hispanic, and 9.5% of other racial/ethnic backgrounds (Appendix Table A). The latter category is heterogeneous, but more granular categories could not be considered because of small cell sizes and unstable estimates. Nearly half had household incomes of less than $50 000. About 88.5% of the sample ever breastfed, and mean breastfeeding duration across the study period was 12.7 weeks among those who breastfed.

In the overall sample and in subgroups by race and income, there was less than a 1% change in breastfeeding initiation, with the exception of decreased initiation among Black respondents (–5.1%) and low-income respondents (–1.9%; Figure 1; Appendix Figures B and C and Table B). In the overall sample of respondents who breastfed, breastfeeding duration increased from 12.6 weeks for births that occurred before January 2020 to 14.8 weeks (17.5%) for those that occurred during January and February 2020. White respondents experienced the largest increase in breastfeeding duration (19.0%). Hispanic respondents experienced the smallest increase (10.3%). High-income respondents experienced a greater increase (18.5%) relative to low-income respondents (16.8%).

The Bayesian structural time-series approach demonstrated that this increase in breastfeeding duration persisted through at least August 2020, before rates dropped to levels consistent with prepandemic trends (Appendix Figure D).

DISCUSSION

This study documents a discontinuous and substantial increase in breastfeeding duration nationwide at the beginning of the COVID-19 pandemic. Widespread shelter-in-place policies were in effect, inadvertently enabling parents who gave birth immediately before the policies to continue breastfeeding instead of returning to work. This suggests a substantial pent-up demand for breastfeeding, which may be stymied by the lack of

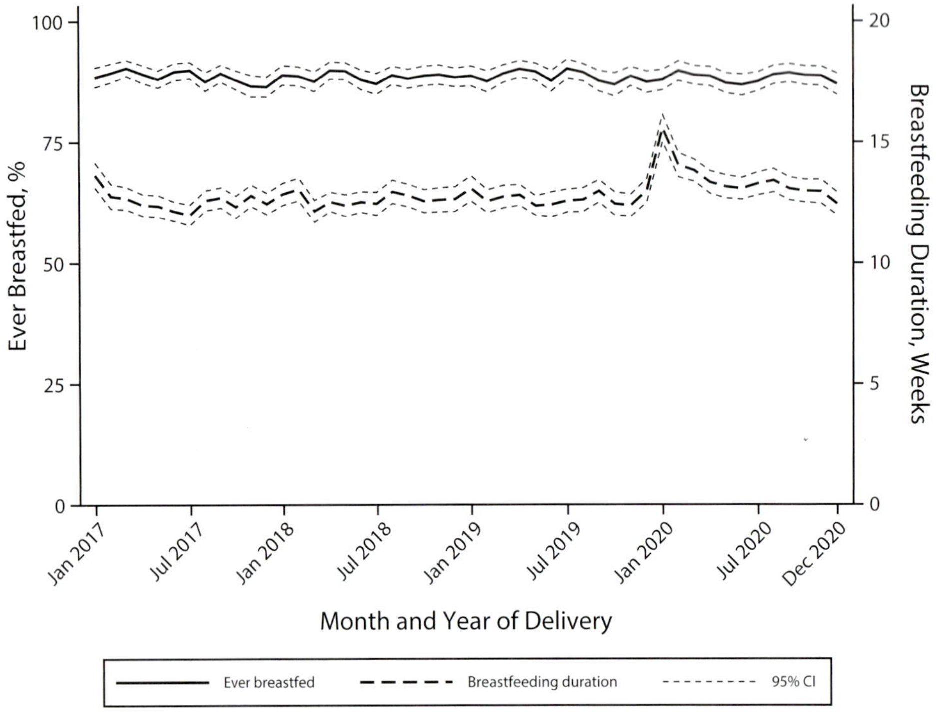

FIGURE 1— Breastfeeding Trends Before and During COVID-19 Shelter-in-Place Policies: United States, 2017–2020

Note. CI = confidence interval. The sample size was n = 118 139 (breastfeeding initiation) or n = 102 518 (breastfeeding duration). Data were drawn from the 2017–2020 waves of the Pregnancy Risk Assessment Monitoring System (PRAMS) and incorporate PRAMS survey weights. The sample was restricted to participating PRAMS sites that collected data on the characteristics of interest during the entire study period.

a national PFL policy in the United States. Indeed, previous work has demonstrated increased breastfeeding after implementation of state PFL policies.[13,14]

At the same time, gains were larger among White and high-income respondents whose jobs could more easily be carried out at home. Gains were smallest among Hispanic respondents who were more likely to be low-wage workers and disproportionately considered "essential" and who already faced structural barriers including lack of paid leave. This may explain the small decrease observed in breastfeeding initiation among Black and low-income respondents. These patterns demonstrate some of the inequities introduced by disparities in the ability to work remotely during the pandemic. When more recent data become available, future studies should examine whether trends and disparities were sustained into 2021 because of new societal norms, the implementation of PFL policies in additional states, or increased remote work during later phases of the pandemic.

Of note, there were no changes in breastfeeding initiation in the sample overall, suggesting that barriers to begin breastfeeding may differ from barriers to breastfeeding continuation. Other interventions may be required to address low rates of breastfeeding prevalence in the United States. The decrease in initiation among Black and low-income participants may be attributable to decreased access to postpartum breastfeeding supports in the context of shelter-in-place.

This work has important implications for the development of a national PFL policy to support the health of parents and infants during the postpartum period. It suggests that rates of breastfeeding in the United States would be higher and more comparable to peer countries if working parents were able to stay home with their infants, and it highlights the need for careful design of PFL policies to ensure equitable access to paid leave. *AJPH*

ABOUT THE AUTHORS

Rita Hamad, Daniel F. Collin, Kaitlyn Jackson, and Deborah Karasek are with the University of California San Francisco. Alison Gemmill is with Johns Hopkins Bloomberg School of Public Health, Baltimore, MD.

CORRESPONDENCE

Correspondence should be sent to Rita Hamad, 490 Illinois St, 7th Floor, San Francisco, CA 94158 (e-mail: rita.hamad@ucsf.edu). Reprints can be ordered at http://ajph.org by clicking the "Reprints" link.

PUBLICATION INFORMATION

Full Citation: Hamad R, Collin DF, Gemmill A, Jackson K, Karasek D. The pent-up demand for breastfeeding among US women: trends after COVID-19 shelter-in-place. *Am J Public Health*. 2023;113(8):870–873.

Acceptance Date: April 6, 2023.

DOI: https://doi.org/10.2105/AJPH.2023.307313

CONTRIBUTORS

D. F. Collin led the data analysis. R. Hamad wrote the first draft of the article. All authors contributed to study design, revised the article critically for intellectual content, and approved of the final version submitted.

ACKNOWLEDGMENTS

This publication was supported by the National Center for Advancing Translational Sciences, National Institutes of Health (NIH), through University of California San Francisco Clinical and Translational Science Institute (UCSF-CTSI) grant UL1 TR001872. D. Karasek's time was supported by the National Institute of Child Health and Human Development and the Office of Research on Women's Health, UCSF–Kaiser Department of Research Building Interdisciplinary Research Careers in Women's Health Program (K12 HD052163).

The authors would like to acknowledge the members of the Pregnancy Risk Assessment Monitoring System Working Group.

Note. This article's contents are solely the responsibility of the authors and do not necessarily represent the official views of the National Institutes of Health.

CONFLICTS OF INTEREST

The authors have no conflicts of interest to disclose.

HUMAN PARTICIPANT PROTECTION

Ethics approval was provided by the institutional review board of the first author's institution (protocol 18-26719).

REFERENCES

1. Victora CG, Bahl R, Barros AJD, et al. Breastfeeding in the 21st century: epidemiology, mechanisms, and lifelong effect. *Lancet*. 2016;387(10017):475–490. https://doi.org/10.1016/S0140-6736(15)01024-7
2. Organisation for Economic Co-operation and Development. OECD Family Database. Paris, France: OECD Publishing; 2022.
3. Meek JY, Noble L, Section on Breastfeeding. Policy statement: breastfeeding and the use of human milk. *Pediatrics*. 2022;150(1):e2022057988. https://doi.org/10.1542/peds.2022-057988
4. Breastfeeding report card. Atlanta, GA: Centers for Disease Control and Prevention; 2022.
5. Chiang KV, Li R, Anstey EH, Perrine CG. Racial and ethnic disparities in breastfeeding initiation—United States, 2019. *MMWR Morb Mortal Wkly Rep*. 2021;70(21):769–774. https://doi.org/10.15585/mmwr.mm7021a1
6. Gyamfi A, O'Neill B, Henderson WA, Lucas R. Black/African American breastfeeding experience: cultural, sociological, and health dimensions through an equity lens. *Breastfeed Med*. 2021;16(2):103–111. https://doi.org/10.1089/bfm.2020.0312
7. Calnen G. Paid maternity leave and its impact on breastfeeding in the United States: an historic, economic, political, and social perspective. *Breastfeed Med*. 2007;2(1):34–44. https://doi.org/10.1089/bfm.2006.0023
8. Bureau of Labor Statistics. National compensation survey: employee benefits in the United States, March 2022. Washington, DC: Department of Labor; 2022.
9. Bartel AP, Kim S, Nam J, Rossin-Slater M, Ruhm CJ, Waldfogel J. Racial and ethnic disparities in access to and use of paid family and medical leave: evidence from four nationally representative datasets. Washington, DC: Bureau of Labor Statistics; 2019.
10. Mervosh S, Lu D, Swales V. See which states and cities have told residents to stay at home. *New York Times*. April 20, 2020. Available at: https://www.nytimes.com/interactive/2020/us/coronavirus-stay-at-home-order.html. Accessed March 22, 2023.
11. Brodersen KH, Gallusser F, Koehler J, Remy N, Scott SL. Inferring causal impact using Bayesian structural time-series models. *Ann Appl Stat*. 2015;9(1):247–274. https://doi.org/10.1214/14-AOAS788
12. Campedelli GM, Aziani A, Favarin S. Exploring the immediate effects of COVID-19 containment policies on crime: an empirical analysis of the short-term aftermath in Los Angeles. *Am J Crim Justice*. 2021;46(5):704–727. https://doi.org/10.1007/s12103-020-09578-6
13. Hamad R, Modrek S, White JS. Paid family leave effects on breastfeeding: a quasi-experimental study of US policies. *Am J Public Health*. 2019;109(1):164–166. https://doi.org/10.2105/AJPH.2018.304693
14. Huang R, Yang M. Paid maternity leave and breastfeeding practice before and after California's implementation of the nation's first paid family leave program. *Econ Hum Biol*. 2015;16:45–59. https://doi.org/10.1016/j.ehb.2013.12.009

CRISPR in Public Health: The Health Equity Implications and Role of Community in Gene-Editing Research and Applications

Andrew M. Subica, PhD

CRISPR (clustered regularly interspaced short palindromic repeats) is a Nobel Prize–winning technology that holds significant promise for revolutionizing the prevention and treatment of human disease through gene editing. However, CRISPR's public health implications remain relatively uncertain and underdiscussed because (1) targeting genetic factors alone will have limited influence on population health, and (2) minority populations (racial/ethnic, sexual and gender)—who bear the nation's greatest health burdens—historically suffer unequal benefits from emerging health care innovations and tools.

This article introduces CRISPR and its potential public health benefits (e.g., improving virus surveillance, curing genetic diseases that pose public health problems such as sickle cell anemia) while outlining several major ethical and practical threats to health equity. This includes minorities' grave underrepresentation in genomics research, which may lead to less effective and accepted CRISPR tools and therapies for these groups, and their anticipated unequal access to these tools and therapies in health care.

Informed by the principles of fairness, justice, and equitable access, ensuring gene editing promotes rather than diminishes health equity will require the meaningful centering and engagement of minority patients and populations in gene-editing research using community-based participatory research approaches. (*Am J Public Health*. 2023;113(8):874–882. https://doi.org/10.2105/AJPH.2023.307315)

AJPH August 2023, Vol 113, No. 8

The discovery and development of CRISPR (clustered regularly interspaced short palindromic repeats) gene editing over the past decade has sparked considerable excitement in the scientific community for its ability to revolutionize the study, prevention, and treatment of human disease.[1] By making gene editing cheaper, faster, more powerful, and easier to use,[2] CRISPR is expected to significantly advance the field of precision medicine by bringing gene-editing therapies to the forefront of health care. However, at present, CRISPR's ability to advance or hinder health equity remains relatively underdiscussed in the fields of population and public health.

Although there is a corpus of excellent literature discussing the potential influence of genomic technologies on health,[3,4] much of this discussion has been centered (1) in the fields of bioethics, education, and law versus health (where it is arguably most needed), (2) on other forms of genomics research and technology (e.g., genome-wide association studies),[5–7] or (3) on the ethics of gene editing on health broadly with limited targeted focus on issues of health equity and disparities[8,9]—with several notable exceptions.[5,10] Also, across thousands of published CRISPR-based studies, few have detailed the benefits and challenges posed by CRISPR gene editing for bridging the health equity gap for minority patients and populations.[4,10]

In public health and medicine, the concept of health equity is grounded in the principles of justice, ethics, and human rights, wherein all people should be valued equally and have sufficient opportunities to live healthy lives regardless of social characteristics, resources, or status.[11,12] Thus, nearly every major US health organization, including the American Public Health Association (APHA), the American Medical Association (AMA), the Centers for Disease Control and Prevention (CDC), and the National Institutes of Health (NIH) have called for research and programs to reduce health disparities and promote health equity for all people.

Under this framework, health disparities are defined as group differences in health status resulting from systemic forms of social disadvantage, such as low socioeconomic status, racism, discrimination, and disability, that increase morbidity and mortality in affected groups.[12,13] Importantly, not all health differences constitute disparities, as disparities primarily afflict minority groups (e.g., racial/ethnic minorities, sexual and gender minorities) because they are disproportionately affected by relative social disadvantage in the United States, leading the CDC to note that health disparities "are directly related to the historical and current unequal distribution of social, political, economic, and environmental resources."[14]

Thus, although CRISPR's emergence has generated considerable excitement in the health sciences, it also raises serious health equity concerns because, historically, minority patients and populations have been persistently excluded from clinical research, innovations, and care—contributing to the current health equity gap by suppressing health benefits for groups experiencing the poorest health outcomes. Similarly, minority participants are minimized in genomics health research,[6,15] as most participants in genomic studies are of European ancestry,[6] suggesting a future patterning in which minority populations will fail to benefit equally from CRISPR advances for improving health. Accordingly, given CRISPR's potential rapid progression from the laboratory to frontline care, the health equity implications of introducing CRISPR gene-editing tools and therapies into public health and health care merits focused discussion based in part on the challenging history of both genomics and medicine in attending to the health needs and disparities of minority populations.[16]

GENE EDITING

Human gene editing refers to the process of making targeted alterations to the human genome using technologies that can modify, insert, or delete DNA sequences.[17] To accomplish this, technologies such as CRISPR employ molecular scissor proteins known as "nucleases" to precisely cut DNA at any site targeted by scientists, allowing researchers to functionally manipulate DNA and alter gene-expressed traits and diseases.[18] Thus, should gene editing fulfill its considerable promise, it may achieve numerous health-relevant purposes, including studying the development and expression of human disease risk factors in laboratory settings and preventing, treating, and curing diseases using gene therapies applied either in human adults or embryos before birth.[19]

Gene therapies (which include but are not limited to gene-editing therapies) refer to biological medicinal products that transfer genetic material (e.g., nucleic acids, viruses) into human cells to alter the human genome for diagnostic or therapeutic purposes.[19] There are 2 categories of gene therapies: somatic and germline.[19] Somatic therapies alter all human cells in the body besides reproductive sperm and embryos and are used to treat existing diseases. Because reproductive cells are not involved, genomic changes made by somatic therapies are not transmitted intergenerationally, reducing long-term risk but also limiting their effectiveness, as they may not reach all cells required to completely treat a disease and cannot reverse prior damage.[20] Ethically, somatic therapies are the least controversial gene therapies and are well regulated, with more than 2000 clinical trials completed or in progress.[21] Thus, CRISPR-based somatic therapies are likely to gain similar public and regulatory acceptance.[8,22]

By contrast, germline therapies target reproductive cells and create heritable gene edits across offspring. Consequently, germline therapies have raised profound safety and ethical concerns with no global consensus reached[8] because (1) any consequences and problems caused by editing may be compounded across generations because every cell in offspring will carry the edits, and (2) these therapies may be used unscrupulously for the purpose of eugenics or enhancing children for advantageous and favorable traits, furthering inequalities.[22,23]

CRISPR

CRISPR refers to short, repeated segments of DNA in bacteria that provide the foundation for bacteria's adaptive immune system against viruses. Specifically, when a virus invades a bacteria, it injects its DNA into the cell, reprogramming the cell to create virus copies until the cell ruptures and releases the replicated virus.[24] If the bacteria survives the attack, its CRISPR system will splice pieces of the viral DNA into the bacteria's chromosome (as short, repeated DNA segments that code for the virus) to create a type of bacterial immunity record.

After a bacteria's CRISPR immune system has encoded a virus into its chromosome, whenever that virus invades the bacteria, the CRISPR system will direct programmable enzymes such as the Cas9 "scissors" enzyme—which can precisely cut DNA at any site like scissors[24]—to locate the virus using specific RNA guides (guideRNA) coded to that viruses' unique genetic signature. Once the Cas9 enzyme locates the virus with the help of the guideRNA, it will bind to and disable the virus by unwinding and cutting its DNA. What makes the Cas9 enzyme remarkable is that the scissors can be easily programmed using different guideRNAs to cut DNA sequences at any gene site. Thus, by combining the Cas9 enzyme with laboratory-designed guideRNAs—creating CRISPR-Cas9 complexes—scientists can edit any DNA sequence in the human body. Impressively, multiple guideRNAs can be employed in 1 Cas enzyme, allowing the simultaneous or multiplexed targeting of numerous genes.

Before CRISPR, gene-editing technologies, such as zinc finger nucleases and transcription activator-like effector nucleases, relied on specially coded proteins to recognize key DNA sequences, requiring complex, labor-intensive development processes that created roadblocks in terms of time, cost, and efficiency (e.g., limited specificity and target recognition, off-target effects).[18] By contrast, by cleverly repurposing the CRISPR system and Cas proteins to cut genes at any desired DNA sequence, scientists can easily target, edit, regulate, and modify the human genome.[25] Through these mechanisms, disease-causing genes can be turned on or off or replaced by inserting donor DNA into CRISPR-Cas9 complexes—allowing researchers to cure human diseases linked to our genetic code.

CRISPR CLINICAL BENEFITS

Because CRISPR can target genetic architectures more precisely than previous gene-editing tools, CRISPR breakthroughs have quickly advanced the health sciences. For example, CRISPR has accelerated the study of genetic models of human diseases by allowing scientists to efficiently induce genetic changes in animal models and study their effects. Through this process, scientists have successfully elucidated genetic pathways for diseases by introducing disease-causing mutations (e.g., cancers) into nonhuman animals, allowing scientists to model human diseases in the laboratory with speed and precision.[1]

Additionally, CRISPR can allow scientists to develop gene therapies to correct point mutations in the genome to treat or cure single-cell hereditary diseases such as sickle cell anemia (SCA), which has received intense research focus as a proof-of-concept application of CRISPR's therapeutic potential.[26] Caused by a single point mutation in the B-globin gene, SCA affects 100 000 people nationally[27] who are primarily of African ancestry or Central and South American descent. Millions of people are also affected by SCA worldwide in Africa, India, the Mediterranean, and the Arabian Peninsula,[28] with available cures involving high-risk stem-cell or bone marrow transplants.[29] Yet, human experiments indicate CRISPR may effectively treat SCA in patients.[30–32] This success provides promising evidence of CRISPR's potential to cure genetic disorders, while also highlighting longstanding disparities in the development of treatment options for minority populations[33] as SCA has historically received limited research and clinical funding[28] compared with genetic conditions that are more prevalent in European ancestry populations.

For instance, despite hemophilia and cystic fibrosis being less prevalent than SCA, large US networks of hemophilia and cystic fibrosis treatment centers provide high-quality specialty care to most individuals with these disorders, whereas only a minority of individuals with SCA receive specialty care[34] owing to limited US funding for SCA networks and centers.[35] Early investments in SCA gene-editing research also raise significant concerns around targeting African American populations in the first CRISPR human trials considering the safety risks associated with previous gene-editing trials[19] as well as concerns involving fairness in application should these trials lead to viable cures given the legacy of discrimination against the SCA community (e.g., denial of education, work, and health care opportunities).[33]

CRISPR PUBLIC HEALTH BENEFITS

The potential public health benefits of CRISPR are murkier as the technology's capacity to influence most major causes of disability and death remain unclear.[2] First, because genes and environment play an intertwined role in many chronic diseases (e.g., asthma, cardiovascular disease), it is questionable whether technologies targeting genetic factors alone can have a measurable effect on health equity, as genes do not appear to be the primary driving factor for many health disparities. Second, because CRISPR therapies operate at the individual rather than population level, any improvements in health outcomes will be limited to a single patient at a time. Yet, despite these issues, CRISPR innovations in disease surveillance, diagnosis, and treatment may someday yield public health benefits if appropriately attuned to minority populations, who bear the heaviest US disease burdens.

For instance, CRISPR may allow clinicians to identify, regulate, and correct certain genetic contributors to chronic diseases (e.g., diabetes, cancer, heart disease) that interact with sources of disadvantage and stress in the environment (e.g., poverty, pollution) to perpetuate health disparities. This includes using CRISPR tools to correct key asthma-linked polymorphisms that increase asthma risk among individuals repeatedly exposed to heavy air pollution[36]—a common environmental hazard disproportionately affecting minority communities.

CRISPR may also enhance public health by strengthening virus surveillance. This is especially true for many low-income minority communities, which often suffer disproportionate rates of infectious diseases caused by viruses such as human papillomavirus, HIV, mpox, and SARS-CoV-2 (severe acute respiratory syndrome coronavirus 2) owing to structural inequities in the social and built environment (e.g., racial segregation, stigma, lack of access to clean air and water, limited health care access). As these viruses are challenging and expensive to track on a population scale using current testing approaches, scientists have developed novel CRISPR-based surveillance platforms such as CARMEN-Cas13: a multiplexed CRISPR-based assay capable of diagnosing hundreds of viruses per sample at low cost.[37] Using CARMEN-Cas13 may allow professionals to efficiently screen people in communities for viruses, facilitating rapid public health responses to mitigate future community outbreaks.

Finally, CRISPR-based tools can be used to address other possible drivers of health disparities, such as poor vector-borne disease control. For example, CRISPR may reduce infectious disease transmission from vectors (living organisms), which cause 17% of all infectious diseases and 700 000 deaths annually worldwide.[38] This ability is illustrated by recent advances in CRISPR gene drives, which can knock out genes in entire populations of disease-causing organisms, allowing genetic modification of vectors at the population level.[24,39] This technology has already been shown in the laboratory to effectively block mosquitoes from transmitting malaria parasites,[40] potentially reducing the spread of malarial diseases that affect hundreds of millions of people worldwide.

Under ideal circumstances, CRISPR may also play a role in combating food insecurity in minority communities and developing nations through the development of CRISPR-Cas9–modified crops (e.g., pest-resistant fruits, high-yield soy and wheat)[41] and livestock (e.g., disease-resistant farm animals).[42] However, given the complex scientific, business, regulatory, and ethical issues surrounding CRISPR-based agriculture,[43] a more fulsome discussion is warranted[42–46] than this article can provide.

CRISPR AND HEALTH EQUITY

From a health equity perspective, although CRISPR may significantly advance science and health care, gene-editing technologies concurrently raise serious concerns about fairness, justice, and access for minority populations. The first concern is rooted in fundamental cause theory,[47] a well-established theory in the public health canon that states that health disparities persist in part because major advances in medicine and treatment overwhelmingly benefit society's advantaged over its disadvantaged.[47] Thus, when novel interventions emerge to reduce sickness or mortality (e.g., COVID-19 testing, vaccines, and therapeutics), individuals with higher social status—who possess greater resources to protect their health (e.g., money, power, knowledge)—have more access to these interventions than do those with minority status, who are often blocked from obtaining equal health-protective resources.[48,49]

Far from being a theoretical concern, many non-CRISPR gene therapies cost between $450 000 to $2 million per treatment,[50,51] with the gene therapies Hemgenix and Zolgensma costing $3.5 million and $2.1 million, respectively, per 1-time treatment.[52,53] These extraordinary costs place gene therapies primarily within the reach of society's most advantaged while excluding much of the population—including many individuals from historically disadvantaged groups who are traditionally denied access to essential social, economic, and health care institutions owing to their minoritized status.[54] Consequently, as novel CRISPR therapies enter the health care marketplace, current inequities in gene therapy access and benefits are likely to worsen because research has linked extreme medication pricing to (1) discriminatory insurance coverage,[55] (2) onerous reimbursement payee issues,[56] and (3) severe copay burdens that create high rates of medication noninitiation and abandonment.[57–59] For example, exa-cel—a CRISPR therapy for SCA expected to receive Food and Drug Administration approval in 2023[60]—is speculated to potentially exceed Hemgenix's pricing because of the $4 to $6 million cost of lifetime treatment for severe SCA.[61]

Beyond cost barriers, minority patients are also less likely to live in communities where cutting-edge CRISPR therapies will be accessible—in part owing to racial segregation—and may have limited knowledge and awareness of these therapies upon their availability. Many of these differences in access, knowledge, and health are heavily rooted in structural racism,[16] which is regularly reinforced in health care through systemic actions such as racially biased doctoring and medical practices,[62] medical abuse in research (e.g., Tuskegee syphilis study),[16] and inadequate or biased distribution of health care resources.[63] Consequently, mirroring calls by scholars at the National Human Genome Research Institute,[5] it is critical that the equitable application of gene editing serve as the bedrock for all research seeking to move CRISPR research into human applications.[5]

Yet, achieving this goal requires addressing a second pressing concern—minorities' glaring underrepresentation in genomics and gene-editing research.[3] This gap is illustrated by a 2016 analysis that found that only 4% of participants in genome-wide association studies were of African, Hispanic/Latino, or Indigenous ancestry.[64] Although recent initiatives such as the NIH's All of Us study have set promising diversity targets, including 50% minority participation, these efforts have received strong criticism for their limited investment in providing meaningful benefits to minority groups for their participation.[65] Accordingly, without meaningfully engaging minorities across all stages of gene-editing research, CRISPR's entry into health care may create numerous health equity challenges.

Initially, CRISPR therapeutics designed without the active research involvement of minority populations may be unlikely to be maximally feasible or effective with minority patients. For example, the Population Architecture Using Genomics and Epidemiology study of 49 839 non-European individuals identified a number of health-relevant complex traits and risk alleles in minority individuals that were previously missed in Eurocentric genome-wide association studies.[7] This poses a concern because genetic architectures in minority and European ancestry populations potentially differ and so may reduce the efficacy of, or increase side effects for, minority patients treated with gene-editing therapies derived mainly from European ancestry samples[7]—thus introducing treatment risks and outcomes that could exacerbate health disparities and intensify mistrust.

Next, given minority populations' warranted cultural mistrust stemming from their historical underrepresentation and unethical treatment in health care and medical research, excluding these groups from meaningful inclusion in research is likely to reduce public acceptance and use of resulting CRISPR tools and therapies. This distrust will likely be especially powerful for DNA-altering technologies such as CRISPR owing to racism's enduring legacy in health care, as demonstrated by many African American communities' strong initial hesitancy toward mRNA vaccines, which triggered antivaccine beliefs and biology-related misinformation (e.g., vaccines cause biological changes affecting fertility and pregnancy).[66,67]

To increase CRISPR acceptance, researchers must therefore cultivate trust in gene editing through transparency and communication, making information accessible, relatable, and culturally relevant for minority groups.[10] However, this leads to a third challenge caused by minorities' limited inclusion in gene-editing research: communicating the benefits of, and combating misinformation about, novel CRISPR tools and therapies to minority patients, who often experience lower health literacy because of language barriers or lack of culturally appropriate health care messaging. To counteract this, health communication research must be firmly situated in the CRISPR research agenda to facilitate minority acceptance[10,68] and establish transparency and trust by identifying (1) their preferred communications strategies and formats (e.g., narratives, community endorsements); (2) culturally responsive and linguistically appropriate images, graphics, and language; and (3) cultural and structural barriers to using CRISPR tools and therapies.[69]

Unfortunately, even when minority groups are included in genomics research, history indicates their contributions can be exploited. In a notorious case, blood samples donated by members of the Havasupai Tribe for a study on diabetes risk were used without their consent by Arizona State University researchers to publish multiple genetic studies on tribal migration, mental disorders, alcoholism, and inbreeding.[70] As these topics were culturally taboo and several findings violated core tribal beliefs and myths, tribal members sued the university, winning a hefty financial settlement to address the harms caused by researchers' misuse of their genetic data.[71] As this case reveals, increasing minority representation alone is unlikely to prevent CRISPR-driven health equity problems from emerging unless researchers engage minority groups as informed power brokers and decision-makers through community-based participatory research (CBPR).

COMMUNITY-BASED PARTICIPATORY RESEARCH

CBPR is a widely accepted collaborative research approach that works to protect public health by equitably involving all partners in the research process—bridging the gap between science and practice through community engagement and social action to promote health equity.[72] According to the NIH, community stakeholders should be fully involved in each research stage from conception to design, analysis, and dissemination, with stakeholders possessing equal voice, power, and decision-making capacity in all project aspects. Through this process, CBPR provides an avenue to reduce exploitation and ensure that minority groups benefit from their participation in gene-editing research, as minority communities are often interested in engaging in ethical research to address their health needs and problems, provided their concerns and voices are attended to in the research process.[15]

Integrating CBPR into gene-editing research carries several key scientific benefits. First, obtaining community involvement can lead to scientifically sounder research by facilitating the recruitment of hard-to-reach or hesitant minority populations into gene-editing studies and by generating findings and data with improved ecological validity. Second, giving minority communities a genuine voice in gene-editing research allows evidence generated through CBPR to be fed back to, vetted, and shaped by community members to tailor and design effective, community-accepted interventions for these groups,[73] increasing the likelihood of intervention feasibility and success. Third, CBPR builds greater trust and respect by stimulating active, participatory dialogue between CRISPR researchers and stakeholders, strengthening long-term research access, collaborations, and direct translation of interventions to minority communities.[5]

To provide a theoretical example of infusing CBPR into gene-editing research, CRISPR researchers studying SCA could engage minority communities as partners and stakeholders in several ways. First, they should approach institutions and organizations in these communities (e.g., churches, cultural organizations, historically Black colleges and universities) to serve as community partners and develop advisory boards consisting of patients with SCA, community leaders, and local clinicians to ensure that community needs and concerns are represented in the research agenda. Second, they should engage these partners and boards in providing feedback and insights on the research design (e.g., hypotheses, sampling and recruitment, analytic plan), coleading data collection activities, reviewing and interpreting results from a community and cultural perspective, and facilitating data dissemination efforts to participants, policymakers, and communities. Third, they should work with partners and boards to develop communication materials containing culturally responsive messaging (e.g., images, terms, narratives) to enhance community acceptance and uptake of ensuing CRISPR products. Although potentially requiring additional time and costs to complete, these efforts are justified by the increased likelihood that CRISPR tools and therapies shaped by CBPR will be more feasible for, accepted by, and effective in minority communities.

Promisingly, some of this work has already begun. In 2017, Persaud et al. engaged diverse SCA stakeholders (patients, parents, hematologists) in research to capture their perspectives toward participating in CRISPR clinical trials.[69] Stakeholders identified multiple barriers that researchers should address to engage patients in CRISPR trials, including fears involving possible complications from trial participation (e.g., infertility, increased disease severity, permanent genomic alterations), the high burdens of trial participation, and whether SCA therapies will equitably benefit their communities.[69] Stakeholders also provided pragmatic recommendations for promoting meaningful research engagement, including engaging SCA stakeholders in designing CRISPR trials; enacting transparency and open access to information about trial protocols, risks, and limitations; having greater community outreach and engagement including partnering with community-trusted brokers (e.g., family physicians); and creating and disseminating patient-centered communications through community-preferred channels (e.g., social media, news channels).[69] Through this work, researchers obtained essential information for promoting CRISPR clinical trial engagement in the SCA community.

Overall, to conduct effective CRISPR-CBPR work, researchers should engage community partners at the start to discuss the purpose, goals, and intended products of the desired research, and develop formal agreements as needed on issues of informed consent, recruitment, data ownership, dissemination, and equitable access to research products. Several Indigenous communities have already developed effective research guidelines, policies, and boards, providing community-supported pathways for engaging these communities—and their valuable genetic participation and data—in CRISPR research.[70,74] Claw et al.[15] have further proposed a framework containing key principles for engaging Indigenous populations in ethical genomics research that includes 4 CBPR principles recommended here that CRISPR researchers implement to perform ethical research with minority groups: cultural competency, transparency, capacity building, and dissemination.

CONCLUSIONS

Given our incomplete knowledge about the long-term effects of CRISPR on health equity and the human body,[4] researchers and funders must carefully consider the ethical and real-world implications of allowing these technologies to be implemented at scale in public health and medicine.[4] If health equity is an essential value underpinning health care and public health, CRISPR research must be made equitable by engaging minority groups as informed stakeholders and decision-makers to ensure that resulting CRISPR tools and therapies are relevant and accessible for populations experiencing health disparities. This includes deciding who gets access to treatments and which diseases are targeted (i.e., selection of investment). However, without appropriate guideposts and mandates from funders and organizations (e.g., NIH, APHA) to center health equity in gene-editing research,[10] it is unclear whether CRISPR developers will focus their investments on treating high-impact genetic diseases that carry the greatest public health impact or merely the most profitable ones.[50]

Unfortunately, neither the APHA's Health Equity Fact Sheets[75] nor the AMA's Health Equity Strategic Plan[76] presently address issues of equity and inclusion in genomic medicine. More positively, the recent Third International Summit on Human Genome Editing[77] encouraged gene-editing equity and access for underserved populations and countries, urging global commitments to advance "equitable, financially sustainable, and accessible treatments" and research that "includes more genetically diverse populations and expanding the range of those who conceive and conduct the research."[78]

Consequently, researchers and community stakeholders should collaboratively develop frameworks and processes to guide CRISPR researchers in promoting health equity through inclusion, community engagement, ethical oversight, and transparency, as it is unlikely health equity will be advanced without strong commitments by all partners to the ideals of justice, fairness, and equitable access in gene editing. However, because the field of equitable genomics remains in its infancy,[5] without meaningful inclusion of minority communities and clear guidelines and principles to assist researchers and health professionals in conducting ethical, community-partnered gene-editing research, innovative CRISPR tools and therapies are likely to result in inequitable access to precision medicine for minority populations—reifying existing health disparities for those suffering society's highest burden of disease.[7] AJPH

ABOUT THE AUTHOR

Andrew M. Subica is with the Department of Social Medicine, Population, and Public Health, University of California, Riverside School of Medicine.

CORRESPONDENCE

Correspondence should be sent to Andrew M. Subica, PhD, University of California Riverside, School of Medicine, Department of Social Medicine, Population, and Public Health, 900 University Ave, Riverside, CA 92521 (e-mail: subica@gmail.com). Reprints can be ordered at http://www.ajph.org by clicking the "Reprints" link.

PUBLICATION INFORMATION

Full Citation: Subica AM. CRISPR in public health: the health equity implications and role of community in gene-editing research and applications. *Am J Public Health*. 2023;113(8):874–882.

Acceptance Date: April 6, 2023.

DOI: https://doi.org/10.2105/AJPH.2023.307315

CONFLICTS OF INTEREST

The author has no conflicts of interest to disclose.

HUMAN PARTICIPANT PROTECTION

No protocol approval was necessary because no human participants or participant data were involved in the development and writing of this analytic essay.

REFERENCES

1. Doudna JA. Genomic engineering and the future of medicine. *JAMA*. 2015;313(8):791. https://doi.org/10.1001/jama.2015.287
2. JAMA Network. Gene Editing Using CRISPR. Why the Excitement? August 29, 2017. Available at: https://jamanetwork.com/journals/jama/article-abstract/2646800?casa_token=pakCcJ9lAjkAAAAA:TK7IHrBDoM3FxtLXDrLWFFKRNq7jL9h5l_oZJ_ftloFW42EBW63THK1_gQlgH7rIUS7HOC1gf94. Accessed December 24, 2022.
3. Hildebrandt CC, Marron JM. Justice in CRISPR/Cas9 research and clinical applications. *AMA J Ethics*. 2018;20(9):826–833. https://doi.org/10.1001/amajethics.2018.826
4. Baylis F. *Altered Inheritance: CRISPR and the Ethics of Human Genome Editing*. Cambridge, MA: Harvard University Press; 2019. https://doi.org/10.4159/9780674241954
5. Jooma S, Hahn MJ, Hindorff LA, Bonham VL. Defining and achieving health equity in genomic medicine. *Ethn Dis*. 2019;29(suppl 1):173–178. https://doi.org/10.18865/ed.29.S1.173
6. Clyde D. Making the case for more inclusive GWAS. *Nat Rev Genet*. 2019;20(9):500–501. https://doi.org/10.1038/s41576-019-0160-0
7. Wojcik GL, Graff M, Nishimura KK, et al. Genetic analyses of diverse populations improves discovery for complex traits. *Nature*. 2019;570(7762):514–518. https://doi.org/10.1038/s41586-019-1310-4
8. Coller BS. Ethics of human genome editing. *Annu Rev Med*. 2019;70:289–305. https://doi.org/10.1146/annurev-med-112717-094629
9. Committee on Human Gene Editing. *Human Genome Editing: Science, Ethics, and Governance*. Washington, DC: National Academies Press; 2017. https://doi.org/10.17226/24623
10. Feliú-Mójer MI. Gene editing communication must center marginalized communities. *Environ Commun*. 2020;14(7):877–880. https://doi.org/10.1080/17524032.2020.1812274
11. Braveman PA, Kumanyika S, Fielding J, et al. Health disparities and health equity: the issue is justice. *Am J Public Health*. 2011;101(suppl 1):S149–S155. https://doi.org/10.2105/AJPH.2010.300062
12. Braveman P. What are health disparities and health equity? We need to be clear. *Public Health Rep*. 2014;129(1, suppl 2):5–8. https://doi.org/10.1177/00333549141291S203
13. American Public Health Association. Creating the healthiest nation: advancing health equity. 2017. Available at: https://www.apha.org/-/media/files/pdf/factsheets/advancing_health_equity.ashx. Accessed March 6, 2020.
14. Centers for Disease Control and Prevention. Health disparities. October 4, 2022. Available at: https://www.cdc.gov/healthyyouth/disparities/index.htm. Accessed December 22, 2022.
15. Claw KG, Anderson MZ, Begay RL, Tsosie KS, Fox K, Garrison NA. A framework for enhancing

ethical genomic research with Indigenous communities. *Nat Commun.* 2018;9(1):2957. https://doi.org/10.1038/s41467-018-05188-3

16. Bhopal R. Spectre of racism in health and health care: lessons from history and the United States. *BMJ.* 1998;316(7149):1970–1973. https://doi.org/10.1136/bmj.316.7149.1970
17. Hsu PD, Lander ES, Zhang F. Development and applications of CRISPR-Cas9 for genome engineering. *Cell.* 2014;157(6):1262–1278. https://doi.org/10.1016/j.cell.2014.05.010
18. Waryah CB, Moses C, Arooj M, Blancafort P. Zinc fingers, TALEs, and CRISPR systems: a comparison of tools for epigenome editing. In: Jeltsch A, Rots MG, eds. *Epigenome Editing: Methods and Protocols.* New York: NY: Springer; 2018:19–63. https://doi.org/10.1007/978-1-4939-7774-1_2
19. Wirth T, Parker N, Ylä-Herttuala S. History of gene therapy. *Gene.* 2013;525(2):162–169. https://doi.org/10.1016/j.gene.2013.03.137
20. Turocy J, Adashi EY, Egli D. Heritable human genome editing: research progress, ethical considerations, and hurdles to clinical practice. *Cell.* 2021;184(6):1561–1574. https://doi.org/10.1016/j.cell.2021.02.036
21. Ginn SL, Amaya AK, Alexander IE, Edelstein M, Abedi MR. Gene therapy clinical trials worldwide to 2017: an update. *J Gene Med.* 2018;20(5):e3015. https://doi.org/10.1002/jgm.3015
22. Marchant GE. Global governance of human genome editing: what are the rules? *Annu Rev Genomics Hum Genet.* 2021;22:385–405. https://doi.org/10.1146/annurev-genom-111320-091930
23. Stein R. Experts weigh medical advances in gene-editing with ethical dilemmas. March 6, 2023. Available at: https://www.npr.org/sections/health-shots/2023/03/06/1158705095/genome-summit-gene-editing-ethics-crspr. Accessed April 4, 2023.
24. Wollert D. The fascinating & controversial new science of CRISPR. *Am Biol Teach.* 2020;82(5):279–288. https://doi.org/10.1525/abt.2020.82.5.279
25. Doudna JA, Charpentier E. The new frontier of genome engineering with CRISPR-Cas9. *Science.* 2014;346(6213):1258096. https://doi.org/10.1126/science.1258096
26. Park SH, Lee CM, Deshmukh H, Bao G. Therapeutic Crispr/Cas9 genome editing for treating sickle cell disease. December 2, 2016. Available at: https://ashpublications.org/blood/article/128/22/4703/101474/Therapeutic-Crispr-Cas9-Genome-Editing-for. Accessed December 16, 2020.
27. Centers for Disease Control and Prevention. Data & statistics on sickle cell disease. May 2, 2022. Available at: https://www.cdc.gov/ncbddd/sicklecell/data.html. Accessed March 3, 2023.
28. Baffoe-Bonnie MS. A justice-based argument for including sickle cell disease in CRISPR/Cas9 clinical research. *Bioethics.* 2019;33(6):661–668. https://doi.org/10.1111/bioe.12589
29. National Institutes of Health. Stem cell transplant reverses sickle cell disease in adults. May 14, 2015. Available at: https://www.nih.gov/news-events/nih-research-matters/stem-cell-transplant-reverses-sickle-cell-disease-adults. Accessed March 3, 2023.
30. Kaiser J. Tweaking genes with CRISPR or viruses fixes blood disorders. *Science.* 2020;370(6522):1254–1255. https://doi.org/10.1126/science.370.6522.1254
31. Frangoul H, Altshuler D, Cappellini MD, et al. CRISPR-Cas9 gene editing for sickle cell disease and β-thalassemia. *N Engl J Med.* 2021;384(3):252–260. https://doi.org/10.1056/NEJMoa2031054
32. Locatelli F, Lang P, Li A, et al. Efficacy and safety of a single dose of exagamglogene autotemcel for transfusion-dependent β-thalassemia. *Blood.* 2020;140(suppl 1):4899–4901.
33. Bonham VL, Smilan LE. Somatic genome editing in sickle cell disease: rewriting a more just future. *North Carol Law Rev.* 2018;97:1093.
34. Smith LA, Oyeku SO, Homer C, Zuckerman B. Sickle cell disease: a question of equity and quality. *Pediatrics.* 2006;117(5):1763–1770. https://doi.org/10.1542/peds.2005-1611
35. Grosse SD, Schechter MS, Kulkarni R, Lloyd-Puryear MA, Strickland B, Trevathan E. Models of comprehensive multidisciplinary care for individuals in the United States with genetic disorders. *Pediatrics.* 2009;123(1):407–412. https://doi.org/10.1542/peds.2007-2875
36. Yang IA, Fong KM, Zimmerman PV, Holgate ST, Holloway JW. Genetic susceptibility to the respiratory effects of air pollution. *Thorax.* 2008;63(6):555–563. https://doi.org/10.1136/thx.2007.079426
37. Storch GA. CRISPR tool scales up to interrogate a huge line-up of viral suspects. *Nature.* 2020;582(7811):188–189. https://doi.org/10.1038/d41586-020-01447-w
38. World Health Organization. Vector-borne diseases. March 2, 2020. Available at: https://www.who.int/news-room/fact-sheets/detail/vector-borne-diseases. Accessed July 20, 2021.
39. Vigliotti VS, Martinez I. Public health applications of CRISPR: how children's health can benefit. *Semin Perinatol.* 2018;42(8):531–536. https://doi.org/10.1053/j.semperi.2018.09.017
40. Adolfi A, Gantz VM, Jasinskiene N, et al. Efficient population modification gene-drive rescue system in the malaria mosquito *Anopheles stephensi*. *Nat Commun.* 2020;11(1):5553. https://doi.org/10.1038/s41467-020-19426-0
41. Molteni M. CRISPR can help solve our looming food crisis—here's how. *Wired.* August 8, 2019. Available at: https://www.wired.com/story/gene-editing-food-climate-change. Accessed July 20, 2021.
42. Singh P, Ali SA. Impact of CRISPR-Cas9-based genome engineering in farm animals. *Vet Sci.* 2021;8(7):122. https://doi.org/10.3390/vetsci8070122
43. Menchaca A, dos Santos-Neto PC, Mulet AP, Crispo M. CRISPR in livestock: from editing to printing. *Theriogenology.* 2020;150:247–254. https://doi.org/10.1016/j.theriogenology.2020.01.063
44. Chen K, Wang Y, Zhang R, Zhang H, Gao C. CRISPR/Cas genome editing and precision plant breeding in agriculture. *Annu Rev Plant Biol.* 2019;70:667–697. https://doi.org/10.1146/annurev-arplant-050718-100049
45. Zhu H, Li C, Gao C. Applications of CRISPR–Cas in agriculture and plant biotechnology. *Nat Rev Mol Cell Biol.* 2020;21(11):661–677. https://doi.org/10.1038/s41580-020-00288-9
46. Lamas-Toranzo I, Guerrero-Sánchez J, Miralles-Bover H, Alegre-Cid G, Pericuesta E, Bermejo-Álvarez P. CRISPR is knocking on barn door. *Reprod Domest Anim.* 2017;52(suppl 4):39–47. https://doi.org/10.1111/rda.13047
47. Link BG, Phelan J. Social conditions as fundamental causes of disease. *J Health Soc Behav.* 1995;Spec no.:80–94. https://doi.org/10.2307/2626958
48. Saegert S, Fields D, Libman K. Mortgage foreclosure and health disparities: serial displacement as asset extraction in African American populations. *J Urban Health.* 2011;88(3):390–402. https://doi.org/10.1007/s11524-011-9584-3
49. Phelan JC, Link BG, Tehranifar P. Social conditions as fundamental causes of health inequalities: theory, evidence, and policy implications. *J Health Soc Behav.* 2010;51(1, suppl):S28–S40. https://doi.org/10.1177/0022146510383498
50. Sherkow JS. CRISPR, patents, and the public health. *Yale J Biol Med.* 2017;90(4):667–672.
51. Wilson RC, Carroll D. The daunting economics of therapeutic genome editing. *CRISPR J.* 2019;2(5):280–284. https://doi.org/10.1089/crispr.2019.0052
52. Tanne JH. FDA approves $3.5m gene therapy for adults with haemophilia B. *BMJ.* 2022;379:o2858. https://doi.org/10.1136/bmj.o2858
53. Wertheimer AI. The world's priciest medicine. *J Pharm Health Serv Res.* 2019;10(3):269–270. https://doi.org/10.1111/jphs.12318
54. Subica AM, Link BG. Cultural trauma as a fundamental cause of health disparities. *Soc Sci Med.* 2022;292:114574. https://doi.org/10.1016/j.socscimed.2021.114574
55. Gruber J. The genetic revolution highlights the importance of nondiscriminatory and comprehensive health insurance coverage. *Am J Bioeth.* 2019;19(10):10–11. https://doi.org/10.1080/15265161.2019.1644822
56. Naveed A, Calderon H. Onasemnogene abeparvovec (AVXS-101) for the treatment of spinal muscular atrophy. *J Pediatr Pharmacol Ther.* 2021;26(5):437–444. https://doi.org/10.5863/1551-6776-26.5.437
57. Gleason P, Starner CI, Gunderson BW, Schafer JA, Sarran HS. Association of prescription abandonment with cost share for high-cost specialty pharmacy medications. *J Manag Care Pharm.* 2009;15(8):648–658. https://doi.org/10.18553/jmcp.2009.15.8.648
58. Dusetzina SB, Huskamp HA, Rothman RL, et al. Many Medicare beneficiaries do not fill high-price specialty drug prescriptions. *Health Aff (Millwood).* 2022;41(4):487–496. https://doi.org/10.1377/hlthaff.2021.01742
59. Doshi JA, Li P, Huo H, Pettit AR, Armstrong KA. Association of patient out-of-pocket costs with prescription abandonment and delay in fills of novel oral anticancer agents. *J Clin Oncol.* 2018;36(5):476–482. https://doi.org/10.1200/JCO.2017.74.5091
60. Stein R. Sickle cell patient's success with gene editing raises hopes and questions. March 16, 2023. Available at: https://www.npr.org/sections/health-shots/2023/03/16/1163104822/crispr-gene-editing-sickle-cell-success-cost-ethics. Accessed April 4, 2023.
61. Liu A. Vertex teases launch plans for first CRISPR gene editing therapy ahead of FDA decision. February 8, 2023. Available at: https://www.fiercepharma.com/marketing/vertex-teases-launch-plan-first-crispr-gene-editing-therapy-ahead-fda-decision. Accessed April 4, 2023.
62. Matthew DB. Just medicine: a cure for racial inequality in American health care. 2015. Available at: https://www.jstor.org/stable/j.ctt15zc6c8. Accessed December 27, 2022.
63. Douglas JA, Subica AM. COVID-19 treatment resource disparities and social disadvantage in New York City. *Prev Med.* 2020;141:106282. https://doi.org/10.1016/j.ypmed.2020.106282
64. Popejoy AB, Fullerton SM. Genomics is failing on diversity. *Nature.* 2016;538(7624):161–164. https://doi.org/10.1038/538161a

65. Fox K. The illusion of inclusion—the "All of Us" research program and Indigenous Peoples' DNA. *N Engl J Med.* 2020;383(5):411–413. https://doi.org/10.1056/NEJMp1915987

66. Hsu AL, Johnson T, Phillips L, Nelson TB. Sources of vaccine hesitancy: pregnancy, infertility, minority concerns, and general skepticism. *Open Forum Infect Dis.* 2022;9(3):ofab433. https://doi.org/10.1093/ofid/ofab433

67. Frisco ML, Van Hook J, Thomas KJA. Racial/ethnic and nativity disparities in US COVID-19 vaccination hesitancy during vaccine rollout and factors that explain them. *Soc Sci Med.* 2022;307:115183. https://doi.org/10.1016/j.socscimed.2022.115183

68. Murphy ST, Frank LB, Chatterjee JS, et al. Comparing the relative efficacy of narrative vs nonnarrative health messages in reducing health disparities using a randomized trial. *Am J Public Health.* 2015;105(10):2117–2123. https://doi.org/10.2105/AJPH.2014.302332

69. Persaud A, Desine S, Blizinsky K, Bonham VL. A CRISPR focus on attitudes and beliefs toward somatic genome editing from stakeholders within the sickle cell disease community. *Genet Med.* 2019;21(8):1726–1734. https://doi.org/10.1038/s41436-018-0409-6

70. Garrison NA. Genomic justice for Native Americans: impact of the Havasupai case on genetic research. *Sci Technol Human Values.* 2013;38(2):201–223. https://doi.org/10.1177/0162243912470009

71. Sterling RL. Genetic research among the Havasupai: a cautionary tale. *AMA J Ethics.* 2011;13(2):113–117. https://doi.org/10.1001/virtualmentor.2011.13.2.hlaw1-1102

72. Viswanathan M, Ammerman A, Eng E, et al. Community-based participatory research: assessing the evidence: summary. 2004. Available at: https://www.ncbi.nlm.nih.gov/sites/books/NBK11852. Accessed July 30, 2022.

73. Subica AM, Brown BJ. Addressing health disparities through deliberative methods: citizens' panels for health equity. *Am J Public Health.* 2020;110(2):166–173. https://doi.org/10.2105/AJPH.2019.305450

74. Hudson M, Garrison NA, Sterling R, et al. Rights, interests and expectations: Indigenous perspectives on unrestricted access to genomic data. *Nat Rev Genet.* 2020;21(6):377–384. https://doi.org/10.1038/s41576-020-0228-x

75. American Public Health Association. Health equity. Available at: https://www.apha.org/topics-and-issues/health-equity. Accessed July 20, 2021.

76. American Medical Association. The AMA's strategic plan to embed racial justice and advance health equity. Available at: https://www.ama-assn.org/about/leadership/ama-s-strategic-plan-embed-racial-justice-and-advance-health-equity. Accessed July 20, 2021.

77. Royal Society. Third International Summit on Human Genome Editing. March 2023. Available at: https://royalsociety.org/science-events-and-lectures/2023/03/2023-human-genome-editing-summit. Accessed April 4, 2023.

78. Royal Society. Statement from the Organising Committee of the Third International Summit on Human Genome Editing. March 2023. Available at: https://royalsociety.org/news/2023/03/statement-third-international-summit-human-genome-editing. Accessed April 4, 2023.

Sexual Orientation and Gender Identity Data Completeness at US Federally Qualified Health Centers, 2020 and 2021

Michael Liu, MPhil, Dana King, ALM, Kenneth H. Mayer, MD, Chris Grasso, MPH, and Alex S. Keuroghlian, MD, MPH

See also Stasenko and Quinn, p. 834.

Objectives. To assess the performance of US federally qualified health centers (FQHCs) after 6 years of required sexual orientation and gender identity (SOGI) data reporting and update estimated proportions of sexual and gender minorities cared for at FQHCs.

Methods. We conducted secondary analyses of data reported to the 2020 and 2021 Uniform Data System from 1297 FQHCs caring for nearly 30 000 000 patients annually. We used multivariable logistic regression to explore FQHC-level and patient-level factors associated with SOGI data completeness.

Results. SOGI data were missing for 29.1% and 24.0% of patients, respectively. Among patients with reported SOGI data, 3.5% identified as sexual minorities and 1.5% identified as gender minorities. Southern FQHCs and those caring for more low-income and Black patients were more likely to have above-average SOGI data completeness. Larger FQHCs were more likely to have below-average SOGI data completeness.

Conclusions. Substantial increases in SOGI data completeness at FQHCs over 6 years reflect the success of reporting mandates. Future research is needed to identify other patient-level and FQHC-level factors contributing to residual levels of SOGI data missingness. (*Am J Public Health*. 2023;113(8):883–892. https://doi.org/10.2105/AJPH.2023.307323)

AJPH August 2023, Vol 113, No. 8

Collecting patient sexual orientation and gender identity (SOGI) data is essential for improving health care access, quality, and outcomes.[1,2] Such data are critical for population health management, furthering understanding of health inequities, and informing interventions to address them.[3,4] Routine SOGI data collection also enables provision of tailored, patient-centered, and affirming care for sexual and gender minority patients.[5] For example, knowledge of SOGI helps guide screening for HIV among most-at-risk populations, such as men who have sex with men and transgender women.[6,7] Disclosure of sexual orientation to providers is also associated with greater patient satisfaction, increased adherence to preventive health measures, and better self-reported health.[8] Given these wide-ranging benefits, the US Health Resources and Services Administration (HRSA) mandated the reporting of SOGI data by all federally qualified health centers (FQHCs) starting in 2016.[9]

SOGI data collection is especially important for serving sexual and gender minority patients at FQHCs, which collectively provide comprehensive primary care to almost 30 million socioeconomically disadvantaged adults and children in the United States.[10] The first national analysis of SOGI data collection at FQHCs reported low completeness in 2016, with missing sexual orientation data for 77.1% of patients and missing gender identity data for 62.8% of patients. A subsequent analysis found that missingness for SOGI data decreased to 36.7% and 26.2% in 2019, respectively.[11] These past analyses, however, have significantly overestimated missing SOGI data because of an inability to distinguish individuals with truly missing data from those who reported "don't know" for sexual orientation and "other" for gender identity.

HRSA addressed these limitations in 2020 by updating its SOGI data collection guidelines to disaggregate these categories.

In this study, we used the most recent national FQHC data to assess SOGI data completeness in 2020 and 2021 and to update the proportion of FQHC patients who identify as sexual and gender minorities. We also evaluated FQHC-level and patient-level factors associated with SOGI data completeness. The goal of this study was to identify remaining gaps in SOGI data completeness after 6 years of mandated data reporting and inform policy and practice efforts to improve SOGI data collection at FQHCs and other health systems.

METHODS

We used data from the 2020 and 2021 HRSA Uniform Data System (UDS), an aggregate data set to which FQHCs are required to submit annual standardized data on patient characteristics. The study sample included 1297 FQHCs that received federal funds under the National Health Center Program through Section 330 of the Public Health Service Act. These FQHCs collectively provided care to 28 108 073 unique patients in 2020 and 29 725 471 unique patients in 2021 from all 50 states, the District of Columbia, and 8 US territories.

Sexual Orientation and Gender Identity

FQHCs were required to report SOGI data for all adult patients (≥ 18 years of age).[12] Although SOGI data reporting for patients younger than 18 years was not mandated, FQHCs were required to provide opportunities for these patients to report this information. Sexual orientation groups included the following: "lesbian or gay," "heterosexual (or straight)," "bisexual," "something else (including queer, asexual, and pansexual identities)," "don't know," "chose not to disclose," or "unknown." Gender identity groups included the following: "male," "female," "transgender man/transgender male," "transgender woman/transgender female," "other (including genderqueer and nonbinary identities)," "chose not to disclose," or "unknown." The "unknown" option indicates that SOGI identities for patients are not known to the FQHC because this information was not collected. All SOGI data were self-reported by patients or by their caregivers if patients could not answer the questions themselves.

Health Center and Patient Characteristics

The UDS contains data on FQHC characteristics, including geography, size, rurality, and provision of services to special populations. Geography in this study was categorized based on the 10 HRSA regions, each consisting of states and territories whose activities are coordinated by a regional office.[13] FQHCs were categorized as urban if their associated addresses were in Metropolitan Statistical Areas, as per the county-level 2013 Rural–Urban Continuum classification system.[14] The UDS indicates which FQHCs receive HRSA grant funding for providing additional services, such as the Ryan White HIV/AIDS Program (RWHAP), Migrant Health Program (MHP), Health Care for the Homeless Program (HCHP), and Public Housing Primary Care Program (PHPCP).

The UDS also summarizes patient sociodemographic data aggregated at the FQHC level. These include the number of patients at each FQHC categorized on the basis of age, race/ethnicity, income level (based on the 2020 and 2021 US Department of Health and Human Services federal poverty guidelines),[15] and being best served in a language other than English.

Statistical Analysis

HRSA granted us permission to access and analyze 2020 and 2021 UDS data, which were stored in a secure Microsoft SQL Server database (Microsoft, Redmond, WA).

We calculated the average proportion of patients with known SOGI data for all FQHCs and at the US state level and presented them on separate heat maps for SOGI. We constructed multivariable logistic regression models to evaluate associations between FQHC-level and aggregate patient-level characteristics and above-average SOGI data completeness. Regression models were adjusted for HRSA region, FQHC size (< 10 000, 10 000–19 999, 20 000–29 999, 30 000–49 999, or ≥ 50 000 patients), age (% of patients younger than 18 years), race and ethnicity (African American/Black, American Indian/Alaska Native, Asian, Hispanic, Native Hawaiian or other Pacific Islander, or White), language (% of patients best served in a language other than English), rurality (rural or urban), poverty (% of patients under 200% of federal poverty guidelines), and receipt of additional HRSA grant funding (RWHAP, MHP, HCHP, or PHPCP grants). We conducted separate analyses using data from 2020 and 2021. Two-sided $P < .05$ defined statistical significance, and we performed all analyses by using *R* version 4.2.2 (R Foundation for Statistical Computing, Vienna, Austria).

RESULTS

Of 29 725 471 total FQHC patients in 2021, sexual orientation was unknown for 8 630 415 (29.1%) patients and gender identity was unknown for 7 122 466 (24.0%) patients (Table 1). Of 21 095 056 patients whose sexual orientation was known, 344 813 (1.6%) were reported as lesbian or gay, 277 585 (1.3%) as bisexual, 16 847 390 (79.9%) as heterosexual, 120 253 (0.57%) as something else, 1 129 357 (5.4%) as not knowing, and 2 375 658 (11.3%) as choosing not to disclose. Of 22 603 005 patients whose gender identity was known, 8 717 558 (38.6%) were reported as male, 12 629 643 (55.9%) as female, 41 772 (0.18%) as transgender man or transgender male, 41 041 (0.18%) as transgender woman or transgender female, 260 487 (1.2%) as something else, and 912 504 (4.0%) as choosing not to disclose.

Across all 1297 FQHCs, the mean percentages of patients with known sexual orientation data and known gender identity data in 2020 were 75.5% and 80.6%, respectively. These mean percentages increased to 76.6% and 81.3% in 2021. Data completeness varied across states, ranging from 59.9% in Massachusetts and 60.3% in Connecticut to 92.3% in New Hampshire and 93.1% in Nebraska for sexual orientation, and from 65.7% in both Massachusetts and Utah to 93.9% in West Virginia and 94.0% in Nebraska for gender identity (Figure 1).

In multivariable models, FQHCs in HRSA region 4 (Alabama, Florida, Georgia, Kentucky, Mississippi, North Carolina, South Carolina, and Tennessee) had higher odds (adjusted odds ratio [AOR] = 1.89; 95% confidence interval [CI] = 1.07, 3.35) than those in HRSA region 1 (Connecticut, Maine, Massachusetts, New Hampshire, Rhode Island, and Vermont) of above-average sexual orientation data completeness (Table 2). FQHCs with a greater percentage of patients under 200% of federal poverty guidelines (AOR = 1.01; 95% CI = 1.01, 1.02) and a greater percentage of African American or Black patients (AOR = 1.01; 95% CI = 1.00, 1.02) also had higher odds of above-average sexual orientation data completeness. The odds of above-average sexual orientation data completeness were lower for FQHCs with 10 000 to 19 999 (AOR = 0.71; 95% CI = 0.52, 0.97), 20 000 to 29 999 (AOR = 0.51; 95% CI = 0.34, 0.76), 30 000 to 49 999 (AOR = 0.48; 95% CI = 0.22, 0.56), and greater than or equal to 50 000 patients (AOR = 0.35; 95% CI = 0.22, 0.56) compared with FQHCs with fewer than 10 000 patients.

FQHCs in HRSA region 2 (New Jersey, New York, Virgin Islands, and Puerto Rico; AOR = 2.07; 95% CI = 1.09, 3.94) and region 4 (AOR = 1.93; 95% CI = 1.09, 3.43) had higher odds than those in HRSA region 1 of above-average gender identity data completeness (Table 3). FQHCs with a greater percentage of patients under 200% of federal poverty guidelines also had higher odds (AOR = 1.01; 95% CI = 1.00, 1.02) of

TABLE 1— Patient Sexual Orientation and Gender Identity Data Reported by US Federally Qualified Health Centers: 2020 and 2021

Characteristics	2020 (n = 28 108 073), No. (%)	2021 (n = 29 725 471), No. (%)
Sexual orientation		
Total reported data[a]	19 470 171 (69.3)	21 095 056 (71.0)
Total missing data[a]	8 637 902 (30.7)	8 630 415 (29.1)
Sexual minority[b]		
Lesbian or gay	310 250 (1.6)	344 813 (1.6)
Bisexual	225 381 (1.2)	277 585 (1.3)
Something else	90 404 (0.5)	120 253 (0.6)
Subtotal sexual minority	626 035 (3.2)	742 651 (3.5)
Heterosexual (straight)[b]	15 190 216 (78.0)	16 847 390 (79.9)
Don't know[b]	1 149 453 (5.9)	1 129 357 (5.4)
Chose not to disclose[b]	2 504 467 (12.9)	2 375 658 (11.3)
Gender identity		
Total reported data[a]	21 014 090 (74.8)	22 603 005 (76.0)
Total missing data[a]	7 093 983 (25.2)	7 122 466 (24.0)
Gender minority[b]		
Transgender man or transgender male	34 151 (0.2)	41 772 (0.2)
Transgender woman or transgender female	32 983 (0.2)	41 041 (0.2)
Other	521 952 (2.5)	260 487 (1.2)
Subtotal gender minority	589 086 (2.8)	343 300 (1.5)
Male[b]	7 927 693 (37.7)	8 717 558 (38.6)
Female[b]	11 513 513 (54.8)	12 629 643 (55.9)
Chose not to disclose[b]	983 798 (4.7)	912 504 (4.0)

[a]Percentages are of all patients.
[b]Percentages are of patients with reported data.

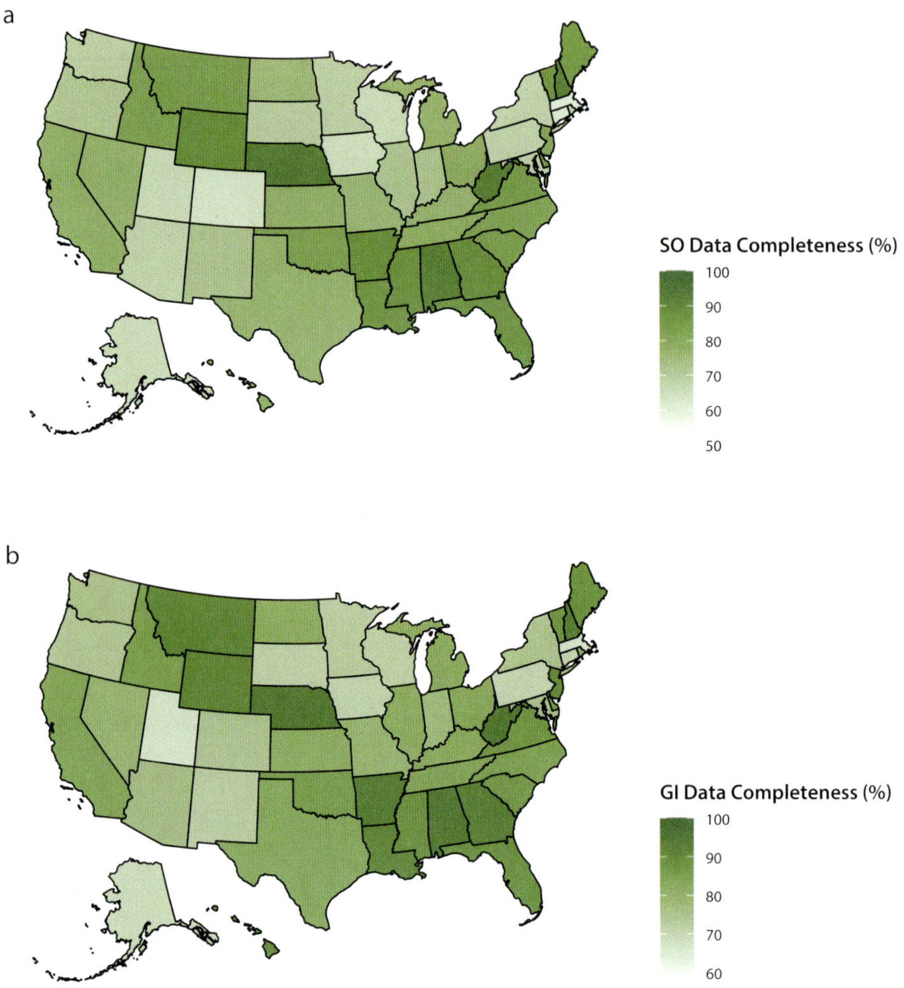

FIGURE 1— Data Completeness by State for (a) Sexual Orientation (SO) and (b) Gender Identity (GI): United States, 2021

above-average gender identity data completeness. The odds of above-average gender identity data completeness were lower for FQHCs with 10 000 to 19 999 (AOR = 0.63; 95% CI = 0.45, 0.87), 20 000 to 29 999 (AOR = 0.41; 95% CI = 0.27, 0.61), 30 000 to 49 999 (AOR = 0.42; 95% CI = 0.27, 0.66), and greater than or equal to 50 000 patients (AOR = 0.31; 95% CI = 0.19, 0.49) compared with FQHCs with fewer than 10 000 patients.

Similar patterns of FQHC-level and patient-level associations with SOGI data completeness were observed in 2020.

DISCUSSION

This national study found that SOGI data completeness at FQHCs increased substantially after 6 years of mandated data reporting. From 2016 to 2021, SOGI data missingness at FQHCs decreased from 77.1% to 29.1% for sexual orientation and from 62.8% to 24.0% for gender identity. These reductions are likely attributable to a combination of factors, including electronic health record requirements to incorporate SOGI data fields, more conducive environments for SOGI data collection, separate categories for truly missing SOGI data, and widespread educational outreach from the National LGBTQIA+ Health Education Center at The Fenway Institute, the HRSA National Training and Technical Assistance Partner tasked with increasing SOGI data completeness across all FQHCs.[16–18] Additional organizations promoting SOGI data collection include the National Association of Community Health Centers and individual FQHCs focused on care for sexual and gender minority populations, such as Howard Brown Health and Whitman-Walker Health.

FQHCs located in the South and those that care for a greater proportion of

TABLE 2— Federally Qualified Health Center Characteristics Associated With Above-Average Sexual Orientation Data Completeness, 2020 and 2021

Characteristics	2020			2021		
	Below-Average Data Completeness[a] (n = 519), No. (%) or Mean ±SD	Above-Average Data Completeness (n = 778), No. (%) or Mean ±SD	AOR (95% CI)	Below-Average Data Completeness[a] (n = 510), No. (%) or Mean ±SD	Above-Average Data Completeness (n = 787), No. (%) or Mean ±SD	AOR (95% CI)
HRSA region						
Region 1 (n = 91; CT, ME, MA, NH, RI, VT)	43 (8.3)	48 (6.2)	1 (Ref)	44 (8.6)	47 (6.0)	1 (Ref)
Region 2 (n = 98; NJ, NY, VI, PR)	46 (8.9)	52 (6.7)	1.34 (0.71, 2.52)	42 (8.2)	56 (7.1)	1.64 (0.87, 3.10)
Region 3 (n = 118; DE, DC, MD, PA, VA, WV)	41 (7.9)	77 (9.9)	1.37 (0.75, 2.50)	45 (8.8)	73 (9.3)	1.21 (0.67, 2.19)
Region 4 (n = 221; AL, FL, GA, KY, MS, NC, SC, TN)	65 (12.5)	156 (20.1)	1.71 (0.97, 3.02)	61 (12.0)	160 (20.3)	1.89 (1.07, 3.35)
Region 5 (n = 187; IL, IN, MI, MN, OH, WI)	90 (17.3)	97 (12.5)	0.82 (0.47, 1.44)	85 (16.7)	102 (13.0)	0.94 (0.54, 1.64)
Region 6 (n = 151; AR, LA, NM, OK, TX)	42 (8.1)	109 (14.0)	2.11 (1.14, 3.93)	52 (10.2)	99 (12.6)	1.44 (0.78, 2.65)
Region 7 (n = 66; IA, MO, NE, KS)	24 (4.6)	42 (5.4)	1.41 (0.70, 2.85)	24 (4.7)	42 (5.3)	1.53 (0.76, 3.08)
Region 8 (n = 54; CO, MT, ND, SD, UT, WY)	23 (4.4)	31 (4.0)	0.99 (0.47, 2.06)	21 (4.1)	33 (4.2)	1.31 (0.63, 2.74)
Region 9 (n = 216; AZ, CA, HI, NV, AS, GU, MP, FM, MH, PW)	94 (18.1)	122 (15.7)	1.32 (0.74, 2.35)	88 (17.3)	128 (16.3)	1.60 (0.89, 2.88)
Region 10 (n = 95; AK, ID, OR, WA)	51 (9.8)	44 (5.7)	0.76 (0.40, 1.47)	48 (9.4)	47 (6.0)	0.92 (0.48, 1.77)
Size						
< 10 000	147 (28.3)	352 (45.2)	1 (Ref)	133 (26.1)	321 (40.8)	1 (Ref)
10 000–19 999	141 (27.2)	234 (30.1)	0.69 (0.51, 0.95)	142 (27.8)	249 (31.6)	0.71 (0.52, 0.97)
20 000–29 999	78 (15.0)	81 (10.4)	0.48 (0.32, 0.71)	79 (15.5)	89 (11.3)	0.51 (0.34, 0.76)
30 000–49 999	74 (14.3)	65 (8.4)	0.42 (0.27, 0.64)	73 (14.3)	74 (9.4)	0.48 (0.22, 0.56)
≥ 50 000	79 (15.2)	46 (5.9)	0.34 (0.21, 0.54)	83 (16.3)	54 (6.9)	0.35 (0.22, 0.56)
% aged < 18 y	26.6 ±10.7	22.7 ±11.2	0.98 (0.97, 0.99)	27.7 ±11.2	23.9 ±11.2	0.98 (0.97, 0.99)
Race/ethnicity						
% African American or Black	16.9 ±21.0	19.8 ±24.0	1.01 (1.00, 1.02)	16.4 ±20.3	20.1 ±24.3	1.01 (1.00, 1.02)
% American Indian/Alaska Native	3.3 ±11.8	1.8 ±7.5	0.99 (0.97, 1.00)	3.2 ±11.8	1.9 ±7.0	0.99 (0.97, 1.01)
% Asian	3.8 ±10.4	2.9 ±8.3	1.00 (0.98, 1.02)	4.0 ±10.6	2.8 ±8.1	1.00 (0.98, 1.01)
% Hispanic	29.6 ±26.8	25.3 ±26.8	1.00 (0.99, 1.01)	30.3 ±27.0	25.8 ±26.8	1.00 (0.99, 1.01)
% Native Hawaiian or other Pacific Islander	1.6 ±9.3	1.1 ±7.4	1.00 (0.98, 1.01)	1.5 ±9.0	1.2 ±7.8	1.00 (0.98, 1.02)
% White	56.8 ±27.9	60.6 ±28.2	1.01 (1.00, 1.01)	57.0 ±28.0	59.5 ±28.1	1.01 (1.00, 1.02)
% best served in a language other than English	22.1 ±22.4	17.6 ±22.0	1.00 (0.99, 1.01)	22.7 ±22.9	17.7 ±21.8	0.99 (0.98, 1.00)

Continued

TABLE 2— Continued

Characteristics	2020 Below-Average Data Completeness[a] (n = 519), No. (%) or Mean ±SD	2020 Above-Average Data Completeness (n = 778), No. (%) or Mean ±SD	2020 AOR (95% CI)	2021 Below-Average Data Completeness[a] (n = 510), No. (%) or Mean ±SD	2021 Above-Average Data Completeness (n = 787), No. (%) or Mean ±SD	2021 AOR (95% CI)
Rurality						
Rural	202 (38.9)	388 (49.9)	1 (Ref)	208 (40.8)	382 (48.5)	1 (Ref)
Urban	317 (61.1)	390 (50.1)	0.74 (0.53, 1.03)	302 (59.2)	405 (51.5)	0.88 (0.63, 1.22)
% ≤200% of federal poverty guideline[b]	56.0 ±25.8	61.6 ±24.4	1.01 (1.01, 1.02)	54.8 ±25.4	59.9 ±24.2	1.01 (1.01, 1.02)
Funding to serve special populations						
Ryan White HIV/AIDS Program Grant	88 (17.0)	92 (11.8)	0.86 (0.59, 1.25)	88 (17.3)	95 (12.1)	0.77 (0.53, 1.11)
Migrant Health Program Grant	79 (15.2)	86 (11.1)	0.85 (0.57, 1.26)	77 (15.1)	88 (11.2)	0.86 (0.58, 1.27)
Health Care for the Homeless Program Grant	109 (21.0)	129 (16.6)	0.94 (0.68, 1.31)	103 (20.2)	135 (17.2)	0.99 (0.71, 1.37)
Public Housing Primary Care Program Grant	50 (9.6)	46 (5.9)	0.70 (0.44, 1.13)	49 (9.6)	47 (6.0)	0.65 (0.41, 1.04)

Note. AOR = adjusted odds ratio; CI = confidence interval; HRSA = Health Resources and Services Administration. The sample size was n = 1297.

[a]Includes federally qualified health centers with average or below-average data completeness.

[b]Based on the 2020 and 2021 US Department of Health and Human Services federal poverty guidelines.[15]

low-income and Black patients were more likely to have above-average SOGI data completeness. One potential explanation is that such FQHCs serve particularly socially vulnerable patients and are therefore motivated and have experience collecting comprehensive data related to demographics and social determinants of health.[19,20] It is also important to note that the ongoing HIV/AIDS epidemic disproportionately impacts sexual and gender minorities and is spatially concentrated in southern states and counties with higher concentrations of low-income individuals and racial and ethnic minorities.[21,22] Thus, FQHCs in such locations are likely aware of their critical role in providing appropriate SOGI-related care to their patients with multiply marginalized and disadvantaged identities.[23]

Despite overall successes, larger FQHCs still face significant barriers with SOGI data completeness and were more likely to have below-average SOGI data completeness relative to smaller FQHCs. This pattern has been observed with data from previous years.[9,11] Larger FQHCs might have more difficulties implementing data collection workflows across multiple settings and engaging a comprehensive range of community-based partners to promote acceptability of SOGI data collection.[18] Such FQHCs could consider established strategies to scale up data collection efforts, such as adding SOGI questions into registration forms alongside other demographic information, incorporating discrete SOGI data fields into electronic health records, and highlighting best practices for SOGI data collection as well as inclusive and affirming care during new staff orientations.[12,24]

It is surprising that FQHCs receiving Ryan White HIV/AIDS Program grants

TABLE 3— Federally Qualified Health Center Characteristics Associated With Above-Average Gender Identity Data Completeness, 2020 and 2021

	2020			2021		
Characteristics	Below-Average Data Completeness[a] (n = 463), No. (%) or Mean ±SD	Above-Average Data Completeness (n = 834), No. (%) or Mean ±SD	AOR (95% CI)	Below-Average Data Completeness[a] (n = 468), No. (%) or Mean ±SD	Above-Average Data Completeness (n = 829), No. (%) or Mean ±SD	AOR (95% CI)
HRSA region						
Region 1 (n = 91; CT, ME, MA, NH, RI, VT)	44 (9.5)	47 (5.6)	1 (Ref)	42 (9.0)	49 (5.9)	1 (Ref)
Region 2 (n = 98; NJ, NY, VI, PR)	34 (7.3)	64 (7.7)	2.48 (1.31, 4.70)	33 (7.1)	65 (7.8)	2.07 (1.09, 3.94)
Region 3 (n = 118; DE, DC, MD, PA, VA, WV)	42 (9.1)	76 (9.1)	1.43 (0.79, 2.58)	42 (9.0)	76 (9.2)	1.27 (0.70, 2.30)
Region 4 (n = 221; AL, FL, GA, KY, MS, NC, SC, TN)	56 (12.1)	165 (19.8)	2.35 (1.33, 4.15)	59 (12.6)	162 (19.5)	1.93 (1.09, 3.43)
Region 5 (n = 187; IL, IN, MI, MN, OH, WI)	84 (18.1)	103 (12.4)	1.04 (0.60, 1.80)	82 (17.5)	105 (12.7)	0.95 (0.55, 1.66)
Region 6 (n = 151; AR, LA, NM, OK, TX)	32 (6.9)	119 (14.3)	3.65 (1.93, 6.89)	43 (9.2)	108 (13.0)	1.73 (0.94, 3.20)
Region 7 (n = 66; IA, MO, NE, KS)	23 (5.0)	43 (5.2)	1.60 (0.80, 3.20)	25 (5.3)	41 (4.9)	1.24 (0.62, 2.50)
Region 8 (n = 54; CO, MT, ND, SD, UT, WY)	19 (4.1)	35 (4.2)	1.49 (0.71, 3.12)	17 (3.6)	37 (4.5)	1.57 (0.73, 3.34)
Region 9 (n = 216; AZ, CA, HI, NV, AS, GU, MP, FM, MH, PW)	84 (18.1)	132 (15.8)	1.97 (1.06, 3.35)	77 (16.5)	139 (16.8)	1.60 (0.89, 2.89)
Region 10 (n = 95; AK, ID, OR, WA)	45 (9.7)	50 (6.0)	0.95 (0.50, 1.82)	48 (10.3)	47 (5.7)	0.77 (0.40, 1.49)
Size						
< 10 000	139 (30.0)	360 (43.2)	1 (Ref)	116 (24.8)	338 (40.8)	1 (Ref)
10 000–19 999	127 (27.4)	248 (29.7)	0.79 (0.58, 1.08)	132 (28.2)	259 (31.2)	0.63 (0.45, 0.87)
20 000–29 999	63 (13.6)	96 (11.5)	0.66 (0.44, 1.00)	78 (16.7)	90 (10.9)	0.41 (0.27, 0.61)
30 000–49 999	61 (13.2)	78 (9.4)	0.58 (0.37, 0.89)	67 (14.3)	80 (9.7)	0.42 (0.27, 0.66)
≥ 50 000	73 (15.8)	52 (6.2)	0.35 (0.22, 0.56)	75 (16.0)	62 (7.5)	0.31 (0.19, 0.49)
% aged < 18 y	26.2 ±10.8	23.2 ±11.2	0.98 (0.97, 1.00)	27.5 ±11.3	24.2 ±11.2	0.98 (0.97, 1.00)
Race/ethnicity						
% African American or Black	17.0 ±21.5	19.5 ±23.6	1.00 (0.99, 1.01)	17.2 ±21.5	19.4 ±23.5	1.00 (0.99, 1.02)
% American Indian/Alaska Native	2.9 ±10.5	2.2 ±8.9	0.99 (0.98, 1.01)	3.2 ±11.9	2.0 ±7.3	0.99 (0.97, 1.00)
% Asian	3.9 ±10.9	2.9 ±8.1	0.99 (0.97, 1.01)	4.0 ±11.4	2.9 ±7.7	1.00 (0.98, 1.01)
% Hispanic	29.5 ±27.0	25.6 ±26.7	0.99 (0.98, 1.00)	28.7 ±26.8	26.9 ±27.0	1.00 (0.99, 1.01)
% Native Hawaiian or other Pacific Islander	1.8 ±9.8	1.1 ±7.2	0.98 (0.97, 1.00)	1.5 ±9.3	1.3 ±7.7	1.00 (0.98, 1.01)
% White	57.2 ±28.1	60.1 ±28.1	1.00 (0.99, 1.01)	56.9 ±28.2	59.4 ±28.0	1.00 (0.99, 1.01)
% best served in a language other than English	22.0 ±22.0	18.0 ±22.3	1.00 (0.99, 1.01)	21.8 ±22.6	18.4 ±22.2	0.99 (0.98, 1.00)

Continued

TABLE 3— Continued

Characteristics	2020 Below-Average Data Completeness[a] (n = 463), No. (%) or Mean ±SD	2020 Above-Average Data Completeness (n = 834), No. (%) or Mean ±SD	2020 AOR (95% CI)	2021 Below-Average Data Completeness[a] (n = 468), No. (%) or Mean ±SD	2021 Above-Average Data Completeness (n = 829), No. (%) or Mean ±SD	2021 AOR (95% CI)
Rurality						
Rural	176 (38.0)	414 (49.6)	1 (Ref)	188 (40.2)	402 (48.5)	1 (Ref)
Urban	287 (62.0)	420 (50.4)	0.72 (0.51, 1.00)	280 (59.8)	427 (51.5)	0.79 (0.57, 1.10)
% ≤ 200% of federal poverty guideline[b]	56.7 ±26.0	60.9 ±24.5	1.01 (1.01, 1.02)	54.8 ±25.5	59.7 ±24.3	1.01 (1.00, 1.02)
Funding to serve special populations						
Ryan White HIV/AIDS Program Grant	77 (16.6)	103 (12.4)	0.93 (0.64, 1.36)	80 (17.1)	103 (12.4)	0.81 (0.56, 1.17)
Migrant Health Program Grant	66 (14.3)	99 (11.9)	0.94 (0.63, 1.40)	70 (15.0)	95 (11.5)	0.83 (0.56, 1.24)
Health Care for the Homeless Program Grant	98 (21.2)	140 (16.8)	0.94 (0.68, 1.31)	93 (19.9)	145 (17.5)	1.05 (0.75, 1.47)
Public Housing Primary Care Program Grant	43 (9.3)	53 (6.4)	0.79 (0.49, 1.26)	41 (8.8)	55 (6.6)	0.82 (0.51, 1.30)

Note. AOR = adjusted odds ratio; CI = confidence interval; HRSA = Health Resources and Services Administration. The sample size was n = 1297.

[a]Includes federally qualified health centers with average or below-average data completeness.

[b]Based on the 2020 and 2021 US Department of Health and Human Services federal poverty guidelines.[15]

were not more likely to have above-average SOGI data collection. Such grants are awarded to FQHCs to support comprehensive health care and support services for uninsured or underinsured patients living with HIV/AIDS.[25] Collecting SOGI data is especially important for the surveillance, screening, and management of HIV/AIDS, particularly given the disproportionate impact of HIV/AIDS on sexual and gender minorities.[21,26]

It is important to note that this study did not specifically assess SOGI data completeness among pediatric patients given the lack of individual-level data. However, it is likely that rates of completeness would be much lower among this population in part because SOGI data reporting mandates did not include those aged younger than 18 years. HRSA should consider expanding data reporting mandates to this population and training providers to ask appropriate demographic questions in a culturally responsive and affirming manner, especially because guidelines are now available to support pediatric SOGI data collection in electronic health records.[27] These data are essential for the delivery of tailored care to sexual and gender minority youths, such as the provision of gender-affirming care and alleviation of minority stress contributing to physical and mental health challenges in this population.[28–30]

Further mixed-methods research and more granular data are needed to identify other patient-level and FQHC-level factors contributing to residual levels of SOGI data missingness. Perhaps more importantly, health systems and policymakers should champion efforts to improve SOGI data completeness across FQHCs, including the development of more tailored outreach methods, a national training mandate, and passage of federal nondiscrimination laws (e.g., Equality Act) that create safer and more affirming environments for SOGI data collection.[31]

Limitations

This study has several limitations. First, the UDS only reports aggregate data, which precludes analyses of individual-level characteristics associated with SOGI data completeness. Second, this study did not assess the role of local-level polices and structural stigma, which are associated with SOGI data completeness.[16] Finally, data were not available to evaluate workforce configurations and the most optimal workflows to promote SOGI data collection. For example, some FQHCs might have more complete SOGI data because of electronic health records that better accommodate structured SOGI data, less organizational complexity, systematic and accurate translation of questions, and internal monitoring to track data collection efforts in real time.

Public Health Implications

To our knowledge, this study provides the most accurate and recent estimates of SOGI data completeness at FQHCs across the United States since HRSA updated data collection guidelines starting in 2020. High levels of SOGI data completeness at FQHCs demonstrate both feasibility of SOGI data collection and success of data reporting mandates. However, there remains a need for tailored support at larger FQHCs, as well as the establishment of broader policies that foster safe and affirming environments for SOGI data collection. These efforts should also be paired with reporting requirements across all health care organizations beyond FQHCs to achieve SOGI data completeness and alignment at a national level.

Moving forward, the increasing availability of SOGI data should be harnessed by health systems and public health leaders to monitor and improve health care access, quality, and outcomes among sexual and gender minority populations.[4] FQHCs could identify specific areas of improvement by stratifying and summarizing quality measures for care experiences, processes, and outcomes in the UDS by SOGI. Progress toward SOGI data completeness must now be met with renewed efforts to identify and address persistent sexual and gender minority health inequities.[32] AJPH

ABOUT THE AUTHORS

Michael Liu and Alex S. Keuroghlian are with Harvard Medical School, Boston, MA. Dana King, Kenneth H. Mayer, Chris Grasso, and Alex S. Keuroghlian are with the Fenway Institute at Fenway Health, Boston. Kenneth H. Mayer is also with the Beth Israel Deaconess Medical Center, Boston.

CORRESPONDENCE

Correspondence should be sent to Alex S. Keuroghlian, MD, MPH, The Fenway Institute, Fenway Health, Boston, MA 02115 (e-mail: akeuroghlian@partners.org). Reprints can be ordered at https://ajph.org by clicking the "Reprints" link.

PUBLICATION INFORMATION

Full Citation: Liu M, King D, Mayer KH, Grasso C, Keuroghlian AS. Sexual orientation and gender identity data completeness at US federally qualified health centers, 2020 and 2021. *Am J Public Health*. 2023;113(8):883–892.

Acceptance Date: April 17, 2023.

DOI: https://doi.org/10.2105/AJPH.2023.307323

CONTRIBUTORS

M. Liu and A. S. Keuroghlian conceptualized the study. M. Liu, D. King, and A. S. Keuroghlian contributed to the design of the analysis. M. Liu conducted the analyses and led the writing and editing of the article. All authors interpreted the data and provided critical revision of the article for important intellectual content. A. S. Keuroghlian supervised the design, implementation, and reporting of the study.

ACKNOWLEDGMENTS

This analysis is based on the Health Resources and Services Administration's (HRSA's) Uniform Data System data. The study authors appreciate HRSA's support of the Health Center Program, including the collection of the data used for this publication.

Note. The findings and conclusions in this report are those of the authors and do not necessarily represent the views or official policies of HRSA.

CONFLICTS OF INTEREST

Alex S. Keuroghlian declares royalties as editor of a McGraw Hill textbook on transgender and gender diverse health care. The other authors have no relevant conflicts of interest to declare.

HUMAN PARTICIPANT PROTECTION

Institutional review board approval was not required per institutional policy because no human participants were involved, and all data were de-identified.

REFERENCES

1. Streed CG, Grasso C, Reisner SL, Mayer KH. Sexual orientation and gender identity data collection: clinical and public health importance. *Am J Public Health*. 2020;110(7):991–993. https://doi.org/10.2105/AJPH.2020.305722
2. Baker KE, Streed CG, Durso LE. Ensuring that LGBTQI+ people count—collecting data on sexual orientation, gender identity, and intersex status. *N Engl J Med*. 2021;384(13):1184–1186. https://doi.org/10.1056/NEJMp2032447
3. Keuroghlian AS. Electronic health records as an equity tool for LGBTQIA+ people. *Nat Med*. 2021;27(12):2071–2073. https://doi.org/10.1038/s41591-021-01592-3
4. Liu M, Sandhu S, Keuroghlian AS. Achieving the triple aim for sexual and gender minorities. *N Engl J Med*. 2022;387(4):294–297. https://doi.org/10.1056/NEJMp2204569
5. Maragh-Bass AC, Torain M, Adler R, et al. Risks, benefits, and importance of collecting sexual orientation and gender identity data in healthcare settings: a multi-method analysis of patient and provider perspectives. *LGBT Health*. 2017;4(2):141–152. https://doi.org/10.1089/lgbt.2016.0107
6. DiNenno EA, Prejean J, Irwin K, et al. Recommendations for HIV screening of gay, bisexual, and other men who have sex with men—United States, 2017. *MMWR Morb Mortal Wkly Rep*. 2017;66(31):830–832. https://doi.org/10.15585/mmwr.mm6631a3
7. Baral SD, Poteat T, Strömdahl S, Wirtz AL, Guadamuz TE, Beyrer C. Worldwide burden of HIV in transgender women: a systematic review and meta-analysis. *Lancet Infect Dis*. 2013;13(3):214–222. https://doi.org/10.1016/S1473-3099(12)70315-8
8. Ruben MA, Fullerton M. Proportion of patients who disclose their sexual orientation to healthcare providers and its relationship to patient outcomes: a meta-analysis and review. *Patient Educ Couns*. 2018;101(9):1549–1560. https://doi.org/10.1016/j.pec.2018.05.001
9. Grasso C, Goldhammer H, Funk D, et al. Required sexual orientation and gender identity reporting by US health centers: first-year data. *Am J Public Health*. 2019;109(8):1111–1118. https://doi.org/10.2105/AJPH.2019.305130

10. Wakefield M. Federally qualified health centers and related primary care workforce issues. *JAMA.* 2021;325(12):1145–1146. https://doi.org/10.1001/jama.2021.1964
11. McDowell A, Myong C, Tevis D, Fung V. Sexual orientation and gender identity data reporting among US health centers. *Am J Prev Med.* 2022;62(6):e325–e332. https://doi.org/10.1016/j.amepre.2021.12.017
12. Grasso C, McDowell MJ, Goldhammer H, Keuroghlian AS. Planning and implementing sexual orientation and gender identity data collection in electronic health records. *J Am Med Inform Assoc.* 2019;26(1):66–70. https://doi.org/10.1093/jamia/ocy137
13. Health Resources and Services Administration. The Office of Intergovernmental and External Affairs. Available at: https://www.hrsa.gov/sites/default/files/hrsa/about/organization/bureaus/iea/hrsa-iea-fact-sheet.pdf. Accessed May 24, 2023.
14. US Department of Agriculture. Rural-Urban Continuum Codes. 2020. Available at: https://www.ers.usda.gov/data-products/rural-urban-continuum-codes.aspx. Accessed August 1, 2022.
15. Department of Health and Human Services. Annual update of the HHS poverty guidelines. 2020. Available at: https://www.govinfo.gov/content/pkg/FR-2020-01-17/pdf/2020-00858.pdf. Accessed August 1, 2022.
16. Almazan AN, King D, Grasso C, et al. Sexual orientation and gender identity data collection at US health centers: impact of city-level structural stigma in 2018. *Am J Public Health.* 2021;111(11):2059–2063. https://doi.org/10.2105/AJPH.2021.306414
17. Ard KL, Keuroghlian AS. Training in sexual and gender minority health—expanding education to reach all clinicians. *N Engl J Med.* 2018;379(25):2388–2391. https://doi.org/10.1056/NEJMp1810522
18. Cahill SR, Baker K, Deutsch MB, Keatley J, Makadon HJ. Inclusion of sexual orientation and gender identity in stage 3 meaningful use guidelines: a huge step forward for LGBT health. *LGBT Health.* 2016;3(2):100–102. https://doi.org/10.1089/lgbt.2015.0136
19. Nath JB, Costigan S, Hsia RY. Changes in demographics of patients seen at federally qualified health centers, 2005–2014. *JAMA Intern Med.* 2016;176(5):712–714. https://doi.org/10.1001/jamainternmed.2016.0705
20. Cole MB, Nguyen KH, Byhoff E, Murray GF. Screening for social risk at federally qualified health centers: a national study. *Am J Prev Med.* 2022;62(5):670–678. https://doi.org/10.1016/j.amepre.2021.11.008
21. Sullivan PS, Satcher Johnson A, Pembleton ES, et al. Epidemiology of HIV in the USA: epidemic burden, inequities, contexts, and responses. *Lancet.* 2021;397(10279):1095–1106. https://doi.org/10.1016/S0140-6736(21)00395-0
22. Fauci AS, Redfield RR, Sigounas G, Weahkee MD, Giroir BP. Ending the HIV epidemic: a plan for the United States. *JAMA.* 2019;321(9):844–845. https://doi.org/10.1001/jama.2019.1343
23. Ard KL, Uzoeghelu U, Bruno J, et al. Readiness of US federally qualified health centers to provide HIV pre-exposure prophylaxis. *Open Forum Infect Dis.* 2021;8(10):ofab447. https://doi.org/10.1093/ofid/ofab447
24. Callahan EJ, Sitkin N, Ton H, Eidson-Ton WS, Weckstein J, Latimore D. Introducing sexual orientation and gender identity into the electronic health record: one academic health center's experience. *Acad Med.* 2015;90(2):154–160. https://doi.org/10.1097/ACM.0000000000000467
25. Cahill SR, Mayer KH, Boswell SL. The Ryan White HIV/AIDS Program in the age of health care reform. *Am J Public Health.* 2015;105(6):1078–1085. https://doi.org/10.2105/AJPH.2014.302442
26. Cahill S, Makadon H. Sexual orientation and gender identity data collection in clinical settings and in electronic health records: a key to ending LGBT health disparities. *LGBT Health.* 2014;1(1):34–41. https://doi.org/10.1089/lgbt.2013.0001
27. Goldhammer H, Grasso C, Katz-Wise SL, Thomson K, Gordon AR, Keuroghlian AS. Pediatric sexual orientation and gender identity data collection in the electronic health record. *J Am Med Inform Assoc.* 2022;29(7):1303–1309. https://doi.org/10.1093/jamia/ocac048
28. Hatzenbuehler ML, Pachankis JE. Stigma and minority stress as social determinants of health among lesbian, gay, bisexual, and transgender youth: research evidence and clinical implications. *Pediatr Clin North Am.* 2016;63(6):985–997. https://doi.org/10.1016/j.pcl.2016.07.003
29. Caputi TL, Smith D, Ayers JW. Suicide risk behaviors among sexual minority adolescents in the United States, 2015. *JAMA.* 2017;318(23):2349–2351. https://doi.org/10.1001/jama.2017.16908
30. Gonzales G, Deal C. Health risk factors and outcomes among gender minority high school students in 15 US states. *JAMA.* 2022;327(15):1498–1500. https://doi.org/10.1001/jama.2022.3087
31. Cahill S, Miller AS, Keuroghlian AS. Sexual and gender minority health equity in the Biden administration. *JAMA Health Forum.* 2022;3(2):e214868. https://doi.org/10.1001/jamahealthforum.2021.4868
32. Liu M, Sandhu S, Reisner SL, Gonzales G, Keuroghlian AS. Health status and health care access among lesbian, gay, and bisexual adults in the US, 2013 to 2018. *JAMA Intern Med.* 2023;183(4):380–383. https://doi.org/10.1001/jamainternmed.2022.6523

COVID-19 Infections, Pandemic-Related Social and Economic Impacts, and Changes to Mental and Self-Rated Health Among Latinx Immigrant Housecleaners in New York City: The Safe and Just Cleaners Study

Sherry Baron, MD, MPH, Isabel Cuervo, PhD, Dhwanil Shah, MPH, Ana Gonzalez, BA, Homero Harari, ScD, and Deysi Flores, BA

Objectives. To estimate impacts of COVID-19 infections and social and economic sequelae on mental and self-rated health among Latinx immigrant housecleaners in New York City.

Methods. From March to June 2021, we conducted a follow-up study with 74% retention of 402 housecleaners initially surveyed before the pandemic between August 2019 and February 2020. We measured rates of self-reported COVID-19 infections, COVID-19 antibodies, and pandemic-related social and economic sequelae and examined predictors of mental and self-rated health changes using logistic regression models.

Results. Fifty-three percent reported COVID-19 infections, consistent with the rate demonstrating COVID-19 antibodies. During shutdown of nonessential services, from March 22 to June 8, 2020, 29% worked as housecleaners, although this was not associated with higher COVID-19 infection rates. COVID-19–related stigma at work, lost earnings owing to COVID-19 infections, housing insecurity, food insecurity, and unsafe homes, including experiencing intimate partner verbal abuse, were statistically associated with changes in mental or self-rated health compared with prepandemic measures.

Conclusions. The disproportionate impact and virtually nonexistent safety net housecleaners experienced during the first year of the pandemic highlight the importance of inclusive stopgap measures to mitigate economic insecurity and its sequelae. (*Am J Public Health*. 2023;113(8):893–903. https://doi.org/10.2105/AJPH.2023.307324)

AJPH August 2023, Vol 113, No. 8

Inequities in the distribution of COVID-19 infection–related morbidity and mortality by race, ethnicity, and economic status are well-documented.[1] Also important to understand is the disparate effects of the pandemic's social and economic sequelae on health. Loss of earnings were potentially significant for many low-income workers and their families, especially immigrants and others who were excluded from unemployment compensation, stimulus payments, and other health and social assistance programs.[2] Understanding these factors can contribute to better public health planning consistent with public health leaders' calls for a new Public Health 3.0 model that more rigorously and effectively monitors and intervenes in upstream social and economic factors linked to health inequities.[3]

To better characterize the extent and distribution of pandemic-related economic and social impacts on health, the National Institutes of Health funded the COVID-19 Social, Behavioral, and

Economic (SBE) Impacts initiative, which provided supplemental funding to ongoing health studies, prioritizing investigators actively engaged with disproportionately affected populations.[4] We report on findings from a COVID-19 SBE study that targeted Latinx immigrant housecleaners in New York City (NYC) enrolled in the Safe and Just Cleaners Study,[5] an ongoing community-based participatory research study exploring the role of working conditions and exposures to household cleaning products on the health of housecleaners, one of the most common occupations for documented and undocumented Latinx women.[6]

We had recruited and administered a survey before the pandemic, between July 2019 and February 2020, to 402 Spanish-speaking housecleaners in the NYC metropolitan area. Results from that survey, exploring pathways through which the housecleaners' employment and working conditions affected their mental and self-rated health, were previously reported.[5] In this follow-up study, conducted between March and June 2021, we resurveyed our participants to (1) document housecleaners' experience with COVID-19 infections and SBE effects during the pandemic, (2) measure changes in the housecleaners' mental and self-rated health compared with findings from our prepandemic survey, and (3) explore how housecleaners' experiences with COVID-19 infections and SBE effects might predict measured changes in the participants' mental and self-rated health.

METHODS

In 2019 we recruited the initial cohort of 402 housecleaners through partnerships with community-based organizations and street outreach in 4 of 5 boroughs of NYC and 2 suburban communities. The prepandemic survey was interviewer administered in person in Spanish, and 70% of those who had expressed interest in the study completed the survey between July 2019 and February 2020. The prepandemic survey participants were similar to the estimated 343 527 housecleaners in the United States in 2019.[7] Participants were 99% female, average age was 44 years, all were foreign-born and had lived in the United States on average 15 years, and only 14% reported feeling comfortable with spoken English. Most were self-employed, worked an average of 22 hours per week for an average of 3 clients, and earned less than $18 000 per year; 44% were the primary wage earners for their families.[5]

For this follow-up COVID-19 study, we attempted to recontact the 402 housecleaners who participated in the prepandemic survey at least 3 times by telephone and text messaging in Spanish to invite them to participate. For those who agreed to participate, a telephone survey lasting approximately 30 minutes was administered in Spanish between March 18 and June 11, 2021, by bilingual or native Spanish speakers trained in survey administration techniques. We collected and managed data using the REDCap tool hosted at the Icahn School of Medicine at Mount Sinai,[8] and participants were offered a $30 incentive.

Of the 402 housecleaners who participated in the prepandemic survey, 296 (74%) participated in the COVID-19 follow-up survey, 27 (7%) were not interested, 24 (6%) had disconnected telephones, and 55 (14%) did not respond. The housecleaners who did not participate in the COVID-19 follow-up survey had similar demographic and employment characteristics before the pandemic as those who participated in the follow-up study except nonparticipants were more likely to report they were the family primary wage earner before the pandemic (59% of nonparticipants vs 39% of participants; χ^2 $P < .01$).

Survey Measures

We measured participants' COVID-19 status using self-report because it was difficult to access medical care or testing in the early months of the pandemic in NYC,[9] especially because 49% of the cohort reported not having health insurance on their prepandemic survey.[5] We measured whether respondents ever had COVID-19 with the survey question "Do you think that you had COVID-19?" or whether they reported ever having a positive COVID-19 nasal swab test. For those reporting they had had COVID-19, we asked whether they had been hospitalized. We also asked the number of household members who ever had COVID-19, whether family members or close friends had died of COVID-19, and whether the respondent had received or planned to receive a COVID-19 vaccination.

Employment-related items captured whether participants worked as a housecleaner during the citywide shutdown for nonessential work (March 22–June 8, 2020), their pay during that period, and whether they returned to housecleaning work after the shutdown. We drew other SBE measures from the COVID-19 resources in the PhenX Toolkit,[10] including COVID-19–related stigma at work, defined as "feeling afraid or embarrassed to tell an employer if they were to have COVID-19" and a 2-item domestic insecurity measure asking whether, since the beginning of the pandemic, the participant felt safe at home and whether they experienced intimate partner verbal abuse. For housing insecurity, we asked about the stability of their current housing situation and the amount of back rent they owed. To assess food insecurity over the previous 12 months, we used the 2-item food insecurity screening tool, which has good sensitivity, specificity, and accuracy in adults, including Spanish speakers and low-income respondents.[11]

To measure changes in mental and self-rated health, we repeated the measures from our prepandemic survey: the Center for Epidemiologic Studies Depression 10-item scale (CES-D-10),[12] Cohen's Perceived Stress 10-item scale (PSS),[13] and the single-item self-rated overall health scale,[14] using the Spanish validated versions of each measure.[15]

COVID-19 Serology Measures

We assessed the validity of COVID-19 self-reports using an at-home self-collected dried blood spot (DBS) kit, replicating the procedures used in another national study.[16] DBS kits were sent from and returned to the study laboratory (Molecular Testing Laboratories, Vancouver, WA) via the US Postal Service in self-addressed, stamped envelopes containing a biohazard bag. A Spanish-language video, developed and validated by another research team[17] and customized with an introduction by our study's outreach worker, demonstrated procedures to complete the home test. We reminded participants at least 3 times to return their kits and offered an additional $20 incentive when kits were returned.

The study laboratory tested DBS specimens for total antibodies using the Bio-Rad Laboratories (Hercules, CA) Platelia test for IgA, IgM, and IgG, which targets the SARS-CoV-2 (severe acute respiratory syndrome coronavirus 2) nucleocapsid protein (manufacturer sensitivity = 98.0%; specificity = 99.3%). The study laboratory also validated this assay for use with DBS, which found 100% sensitivity and 100% specificity.[18] Participants received letters from a study physician explaining their results.

Data Analysis

After conducting descriptive analyses, we compared demographic, employment-related, and social characteristics of those who reported having had COVID-19 to these characteristics of those who did not by using the χ^2 test for categorical variables or the *t* test for continuous variables. We next examined predictors of depression (CES-D-10), perceived stress (PSS), and self-rated health using separate logistic regression models for each outcome measure. To dichotomize these outcome measures, we used the same cutpoints as in our prepandemic study.[5] For the CES-D-10, we used the recommended cutpoint (≥ 10).[19] For the PSS, we used a cutpoint suggested for health screenings (≥ 14)[20] and consistent with the mean score found in the Hispanic Community Health Study.[15] For self-rated health, we compared those reporting poor or fair health to those reporting good, very good, or excellent health.

Our modeling used a stepwise elimination method in multiple stages beginning with demographic and COVID-19–related variables, then employment-related variables, then other SBE variables. At each step, we retained variables significant at $\alpha = 0.2$. In the final step, we added the baseline prepandemic value of the health outcome being modeled and retained all variables significant at the $\alpha = 0.05$ level. We estimated adjusted odds ratios (AORs) along with 95% confidence intervals (CIs). We dichotomized predictor variables unless otherwise specified. To differentiate the magnitude of food insecurity, we created an ordinal scale (0–4) by summing the 2 responses, with "sometimes" experiencing food insecurity contributing 1 point and "often" contributing 2 points for each of the questions. We excluded participants with missing information on a variable only from analyses involving that variable. We conducted all analyses using SAS version 9.2 (SAS Institute, Cary, NC).

RESULTS

At the time of the survey, 153 participants (51.7%) reported that they had ever had COVID-19, and of those, 9 (5.9%) reported being hospitalized. The seasonal distribution of cases (spring 2020: 55%; summer and fall 2020: 16%; and winter 2021: 29%) mirrored the overall pattern in NYC.[21] Among those who did not think or did not know whether they had COVID-19, 5 participants (1.7%) reported a positive nasal swab test. Of the 296 participants, 218 (74%) consented to receive a DBS kit, and 116 (53% of those receiving a kit and 39% of survey participants) returned their kit. The rate of self-reported COVID-19 was similar between those who returned the DBS kit and the others (Table 1). Of the 116 returned samples, only 5 (4%) were indeterminant and 66 (57%) were positive for antibodies. Among those with positive antibodies, 18% reported not having had COVID-19, and 27% of those reporting having had COVID-19 tested negative for antibodies (Table 1).

TABLE 1— **Self-Reports of COVID-19 Infections and Dry Blood Spot (DBS) SARS-CoV-2 Antibody Home Testing Results: Safe and Just Cleaners Study, New York City, March–June 2021**

Self-Report of Ever Having Had COVID-19	All Participants (n = 296), No. (%)	Returned DBS Kit (n = 116), No. (%)	Antibody Positive DBS Results (n = 66), No. (%)	Antibody Negative DBS Results (n = 45), No. (%)	Antibody Indeterminant DBS Results (n = 5), No. (%)
Yes	158[a] (53)	63[b] (54)	49[b] (74)	12 (27)	2 (40)
Don't Know	21 (7)	8 (7)	5 (8)	3 (7)	0 (0)
No	117 (40)	45 (39)	12 (18)	30 (67)	3 (60)

Note. SARS-Cov-2 = severe acute respiratory syndrome coronavirus 2.

[a]Includes 5 participants who reported positive COVID-19 nasal swab tests and "no" (n = 4) or "prefer not to answer" (n = 1) when asked whether they had had COVID-19.

[b]Includes 1 participant who reported a positive COVID-19 nasal swab test but answered "prefer not to answer" when asked whether they had had COVID-19.

Impacts

Table 2 provides descriptive statistics for COVID-19 infection–related and SBE effects. COVID-19 deaths among family members and close friends were reported by 152 (51%) of participants. Participant acceptance of the COVID-19 vaccine appeared high. The vaccine became available to all adults in NYC at the beginning of April 2021. During the first half of our survey administration period, March 18 to April 30, 2021, only 27% (n = 44) had received at least 1 COVID-19 vaccine shot. For those surveyed between May 1 and June 11, 66% (n = 88) reported receiving at least 1 shot. Most (76%) of those not vaccinated intended to get vaccinated.

Most participants (93%; n = 275) reported they were still working in housecleaning in March 2020 just before the citywide COVID-19 shutdown period (March 22–June 8, 2020), and of those, 85 (31%) continued to work as housecleaners during the shutdown, 144 (52%) reported not receiving any housecleaning income during the shutdown, and 43 (16%) reported losing paid housecleaning workdays because they were concerned they might infect their client (Table 2). Many housecleaners who reported losing pay during the shutdown because they were concerned they might infect their client likely lost pay because they themselves had COVID-19. Among those who lost paid workdays during the spring 2020 shutdown period, 23 (53%) reported having had COVID-19 during spring 2020 compared with 61 (24%) of all other study participants ($P < .01$).

At the end of the shutdown, 231 participants (78%) worked as housecleaners, 17 (6%) worked in a job other than housecleaning, and 48 (16%) were not employed. For the working housecleaners, 128 (55%) reported they were extremely or very concerned about having enough clients to meet their financial needs. We also found that only 84 (36%) felt they could take sick leave, paid or unpaid, during the pandemic without retaliation. Given widespread concern about infection control, 142 (61%) reported using more disinfectant cleaning products at work. Almost half of all respondents (47%; n = 138) reported that if diagnosed with COVID-19, they would be likely or somewhat likely to feel afraid or embarrassed to disclose this information to their employer.

At the time of the survey, March to June 2021, most respondents (89%; n = 265) were employed, yet 207 (70%) reported earning less than $1000 per month from all jobs, and 133 (45%) reported being their family's primary wage earner. Since March 2020, only 8% (n = 23) of all participants had received unemployment compensation, 32% (n = 94) received Supplemental Nutrition Assistance, and 11% (n = 34) had received any other form of governmental financial benefits.

Given such low earnings and benefits, it is unsurprising that reports of food insecurity were common, with 254 (86%) indicating they "sometimes" or "often" experience food insecurity on at least 1 of the 2 food insecurity questions. Housing insecurity was also common. Although only 16 participants (5%) did not have a fixed place to live, 118 (40%) worried about having a secure living situation in the future, and 71 (24%) reported being behind on rent by at least $1000. Regarding domestic safety, excluding 7 participants who did not feel comfortable answering these questions, 59 (20%) reported feeling only a little safe or unsafe inside their own

TABLE 2— COVID-19–Related Impacts; Employment, Social, and Economic Impacts; and Mental and Self-Rated Health: Safe and Just Cleaners Study, New York City, March–June 2021

	No. (%)
COVID-19–related impacts	
Infection and exposure	
Self-reported ever had COVID-19 or a positive test	158[a] (53)
Hospitalized with COVID-19	9 (3)
Not hospitalized but had COVID-19	149 (50)
Other members of household ever had COVID-19	182 (61)
Family/friends in US or other country died of COVID-19	152 (51)
Vaccination status	
Vaccinated with at least 1 COVID-19 shot	132 (45)
Among 163 surveys completed March 18–April 30	44 (27)
Among 133 surveys completed May 1–June 11	88 (66)
Not vaccinated but probably will get vaccinated	123 (42)
Employment-related impacts	
Still worked as a housecleaner in February 2020	275 (93)
Worked as housecleaner during March–June 2020 shutdown	85 (31)
Lost paid work days during shutdown because they might infect their client	43 (16)
Did not work and received no compensation from clients during shutdown	144 (52)
Worked as housecleaner after the end of the shutdown in June 2020	231 (78)
Could take sick leave (paid or unpaid) during pandemic without retaliation	84 (36)
Extremely/very concerned about having enough clients to meet needs	128 (55)
Used more disinfectant cleaning products at work after the shutdown	142 (61)
If diagnosed with COVID-19, would be likely/somewhat likely to feel afraid or embarrassed to disclose this information to your employer	138 (47)
Among those who reported having COVID-19	75 (49)
Among those who reported not having COVID-19	63 (44)
Earning per month from all jobs at time of the survey, $	
Not working	31 (11)
≤ 500	120 (41)
500–1000	87 (29)
≥ 1000	45 (15)
Received governmental financial benefits since March 2020	
Unemployment compensation	23 (8)
Supplemental nutrition assistance benefits	94 (32)
Any other government assistance	34 (11)
Food insecurity, in the past 12 mo	
Q1. Worried your food would run out before you had money to buy more	
Sometimes	138 (47)
Often	102 (34)
Q2. The food you bought did not last and you didn't have money to buy more	
Sometimes	152 (51)
Often	61 (21)
Responding "sometimes" or "often" to Q1 or Q2	254 (86)
Other social and economic impacts	
Housing insecurity	
Does not have a fixed place to live	16 (5)

Continued

TABLE 2— Continued

	No. (%)
Currently has a place to stay but worries about the future	118 (40)
Owes more than $1000 in back rent	71 (24)
Domestic insecurity since the pandemic began[b]	
Q1. Level of feeling safe inside their own home (only a little safe/unsafe)	59 (20)
Q2. Someone with whom they had romantic relationships yelled at them or said things that made them feel scared or bad about themselves?	35 (12)
Either Q1 or Q2 (but not both)	86 (30)
Mental and self-rated health outcomes	
Depression (CES-D 10 ≥ 10)	
Prepandemic survey	65 (22)
During pandemic survey	100 (34)
New onset since prepandemic survey	59 (20)
Moderate/high perceived stress (Cohen's PSS ≥ 14)	
Prepandemic survey	130 (44)
During pandemic survey	160 (54)
New onset since prepandemic survey	63 (21)
Fair/poor self-rated health	
Prepandemic survey	86 (29)
During pandemic survey	129 (44)
New onset since prepandemic survey	68 (23)

Note. PSS = Perceived Stress 10-item scale. Study sample size was n = 296.

[a]Includes 5 participants who reported positive COVID-19 nasal swab tests and "no" (n = 4) or "prefer not to answer" (n = 1) when asked whether they had COVID-19.

[b]This excludes 7 participants who did not feel comfortable responding to questions about the safety of their home.

home, 35 (12%) reported verbal abuse from a romantic partner, and 86 participants (30%) reported at least 1 of these aspects of domestic insecurity.

Mental and Self-Rated Health Measures

Compared with prepandemic responses, more participants exceeded the threshold cutpoint for the mental and self-rated health measures. We found that 20%, 21%, and 23% of participants formerly below the cutpoint exceeded the cutpoint on the follow-up survey for depression, perceived stress, and fair or poor self-rated health, respectively (Table 2).

Socioeconomic Conditions and COVID-19

We examined whether employment status, living conditions, or demographic characteristics were related to a respondent's having had COVID-19. When comparing housecleaners reporting COVID-19 or a positive test to others in the study, the only difference found was in the likelihood of living with household members who also had had COVID-19: 89% of those reporting COVID-19 versus 30% of others (Table 3).

Predictors

Multivariable logistic regression models for depression, perceived stress, and fair or poor self-rated health, adjusting for prepandemic measures, found increased odds associated with COVID-19 and SBE-related factors (Table 4). In the fully adjusted models, we found increased odds for depression for those reporting COVID-19 (OR = 1.95; 95% CI = 1.10, 3.45 for nonhospitalized participants; OR = 5.09; 95% CI = 0.91, 28.36 for hospitalized participants). We also found increased odds for perceived stress among those not yet vaccinated (OR = 2.39; 95% CI = 1.28, 4.45), those with household members who had COVID-19 (OR = 1.93; 95% CI = 1.04, 3.60), and those with family members or close friends who died of COVID-19 (OR = 1.84; 95% CI = 1.01, 3.35).

TABLE 3— Self-Reported COVID-19 Status by Demographic, Social, and Employment Conditions: Safe and Just Cleaners Study, New York City, March–June 2021

	Ever Had COVID-19[a] (n = 158), Mean ± SD or No. (%)	Did Not Have COVID-19 (n = 138), Mean ± SD or No. (%)	*P*[b]
Age, y	44.9 ± 9.7	44.7 ± 9.9	.88
Years living in United States	17.4 ± 8.5	16.1 ± 9.5	.21
Education level			.5
Primary school	50 (31.7)	35 (25.4)	
High school	74 (46.8)	61 (44.2)	
General equivalency diploma	5 (3.2)	6 (4.4)	
At least some college	29 (18.4)	36 (26.1)	
English comfort			.38
Uncomfortable	60 (38)	49 (36.3)	
More or less	78 (49.4)	61 (45.2)	
Comfortable	20 (12.7)	25 (18.5)	
Primary family wage earner			.89
Yes	61 (38.6)	54 (39.4)	
No	97 (61.4)	83 (60.6)	
Health insurance			.73
Yes	72 (45.6)	69 (50)	
No	84 (53.2)	67 (48.6)	
Don't know	2 (1.3)	2 (1.5)	
No. of people in household with COVID-19			.001
0	18 (11.4)	96 (69.6)	
1	33 (20.9)	21 (15.2)	
2	35 (22.2)	5 (3.6)	
3	32 (20.3)	9 (6.5)	
≥ 4	40 (25.2)	7 (5.1)	
Asked to work during COVID-19 shutdown (March–June 2020)[c]			.29
Yes	41 (27.5)	44 (34.9)	
No	107 (71.8)	82 (65.1)	
Don't know	1 (0.7)	0	
Employment in housecleaning after end of the shutdown in June 2020			.2
Worked continuously	22 (13.9)	30 (21.7)	
Worked on and off	101 (63.9)	78 (56.5)	
Stopped working in housecleaning	35 (22.2)	30 (21.7)	

[a]We defined reported COVID-19 as self-reporting ever having had COVID-19 or a positive nasal swab test for COVID-19 at the time of the survey: March–June 2021.
[b]*P* value for continuous variables from the *t* test and for categorical variables from the χ^2 test.
[c]This variable includes only those still working as housecleaners in March 2020, right before the shutdown (n = 275).

Regarding employment-related factors, we found increased odds for perceived stress among those likely or somewhat likely to feel afraid or embarrassed to tell their employer whether they had COVID-19 (OR = 3.09; 95% CI = 1.71, 5.58). We found increased odds for fair or poor self-rated health for those reporting having lost wages during the pandemic shutdown owing to housecleaners' concern that they might infect their clients (OR = 2.21; 95% CI = 1.05, 4.69).

Regarding other SBE effects, we found increased odds for perceived

TABLE 4— COVID-19 Infection-Related and Social and Economic Impacts Predictors of Perceived Stress, Depression, and Self-Rated Health: Safe and Just Cleaners Study, New York City, March–June 2021

	Moderate/Severe Perceived Stress (PSS ≥ 14), OR (95% CI)	Depression (CES-D 10 ≥ 10), OR (95% CI)	Poor/Fair Self-Rated Health,[a] OR (95% CI)
COVID-19 infection-related impacts			
Household member COVID-19 status			
≥ 1 member had COVID-19	1.93 (1.04, 3.60)	NA	NA
No member had COVID-19	1 (Ref)		
COVID-19 deaths of family/close friends			
Experienced deaths	1.84 (1.01, 3.35)	NA	NA
Did not experience deaths	1 (Ref)		
COVID-19 vaccination status			
Not yet vaccinated	2.39 (1.28, 4.45)	NA	NA
≥ 1 vaccine shot	1 (Ref)		
Self-reported COVID-19 disease			
Hospitalized with COVID-19	NA	5.09 (0.91, 28.36)	NA
Had COVID-19 but not hospitalized [a]		1.95 (1.10, 3.45)	
Didn't have/don't know		1 (Ref)	
Employment-related impacts			
Would feel afraid or embarrassed to disclose to employer whether they had COVID-19			
Likely/somewhat likely	3.09 (1.71, 5.58)	NA	NA
Somewhat unlikely/unlikely	1 (Ref)		
Pay during shutdown			
Lost housecleaning pay during shutdown because respondent might infect client with COVID-19[a]	NA	NA	2.21 (1.05, 4.69)
Did not work during shutdown or if worked, did not lose pay because respondent might infect client			1 (Ref)
Other social and economic impacts			
Food insecurity[b]			
Yes	1.35 (1.05, 1.73)	1.46 (1.15, 1.84)	1.57 (1.23, 2.00)
No	1 (Ref)	1 (Ref)	1 (Ref)
Domestic insecurity			
Unsafe/a little unsafe and/or experienced IP verbal abuse	2.04 (1.06, 3.91)	2.12 (1.17, 3.83)	2.11 (1.14, 3.89)
Felt safe and no IP verbal abuse	1 (Ref)	1 (Ref)	1 (Ref)
Housing insecurity		NA	NA
No fixed home/worried about future	1.83 (1.01, 3.33)		
Had a stable place to live	1 (Ref)		
Prepandemic mental and self-rated health[c]			
Perceived stress (PSS ≥ 14)	4.40 (2.41, 8.02)	NA	NA
Depressed (CES-D 10 ≥ 10)	NA	3.42 (1.78, 6.58)	NA
Poor/fair self-rated health	NA	NA	5.09 (2.70, 9.59)

Note. CES-D 10 = Center for Epidemiologic Studies Depression 10-item scale; CI = confidence interval; IP = intimate partner; NA = variable not included in the final model because it was eliminated in the stepwise regression analysis; OR = odds ratio; PSS = Cohen's Perceived Stress scale. We adjusted all models for age, educational attainment, and whether the participants indicated they were the primary family wage earner in their prepandemic survey. We included the prepandemic mental and self-rated health variables in the models only for that same outcome measure.

[a]Models containing this variable included only the 275 housecleaners who were still working in housecleaning in March 2020 because those no longer working were not asked this question.

[b]4-point food insecurity scale: 1 point each for answering "sometimes" on the 2-item food insecurity measure, 2 points each for answering "often," reference is answering no to both questions.

[c]We collected all prepandemic measures between August 2019 and February 2020.

stress for those reporting no fixed place to live or worry about future housing (OR = 1.83; 95% CI = 1.01, 3.33). We found increased odds for those reporting food insecurity (OR = 1.35; 95% CI = 1.05, 1.73 for perceived stress; OR = 1.46; 95% CI = 1.15, 1.84 for depression; and OR = 1.57; 95% CI = 1.23, 2.00 for self-rated health). Similarly, those experiencing domestic insecurity had increased odds for all 3 outcomes (OR = 2.04; 95% CI = 1.06, 3.91 for perceived stress; OR = 2.12; 95% CI = 1.17, 3.83 for depression; and OR = 2.11; 95% CI = 1.14, 3.89 for self-rated health).

DISCUSSION

Our study provides insight into the health and well-being of a sample of Latinx immigrant housecleaners in NYC at the beginning of the second year of the COVID-19 pandemic (March–June 2021), and we were able to compare mental and self-rated health measures to measures collected in the 6 months before the pandemic-related shutdown in NYC. Our findings contribute to the literature by providing a unique and comprehensive picture of the depth of the pandemic's impact on a population of workers who faced a multitude of disproportionate risks.

We found that 53% of our participants reported ever having had COVID-19 before being surveyed between March 18 and June 11, 2021, and this high rate of infection was confirmed by COVID-19 antibody tests. The housecleaners' rate of infection was almost double the rate documented over a similar period in a national COVID-19 seroprevalence study of blood donors[22] and is consistent with previous estimates of the increased risk of infection among immigrant Latinx populations, especially in the first year of the pandemic.[1]

Almost one third reported working as housecleaners during the shutdown of nonessential work, from March 22 to June 8, 2020, although we did not find that this was associated with higher rates of reported COVID-19 infections. We also documented a myriad of other SBE effects, including reduced employment and low earnings, perceived COVID-19–related stigma at work, food and housing insecurity, and feeling unsafe at home or experiencing intimate partner verbal abuse. As has been widely reported in other studies,[23] we found deterioration in housecleaners' mental and self-rated health compared with prepandemic levels, with COVID-19 infection, employment, and other SBE impacts contributing. Lastly, although studies have found mixed results related to vaccine acceptance among Latinx populations,[24] our findings suggest a high level of acceptance.

Our findings are consistent with other COVID-19 studies that included larger and more diverse populations. For example, a national survey found that all racial and ethnic minorities— but especially those having limited English proficiency, less education, and lower incomes and those living in large cities—were more likely to report that people acted afraid of them because of suspected COVID-19 infection.[25] A national food insecurity study using the same 2-item measure found an increased risk of food insecurity among Hispanic and low-income populations and also found associations between becoming food insecure and anxiety and depression.[26] A national sample of US adults found that housing insecurity, defined as being afraid of being behind on rent or mortgage payments, was associated with higher psychological distress and lower self-rated health during the COVID-19 pandemic.[27]

Fewer studies have examined COVID-19–related risks associated with domestic safety and intimate partner abuse because of challenges in collecting such data,[28] although public health experts have highlighted the potential risks.[29] Finally, the rates of employment, housing, and food insecurity documented in our study are consistent with findings from a national survey of Spanish-speaking domestic workers conducted by the National Domestic Workers Alliance during the first 6 months of the pandemic.[30] Our study adds to these previous studies by capturing how multifaceted SBE stressors together with the direct effects of COVID-19 infections contributed to changes in mental and self-rated health in our sample of Latinx immigrant housecleaners in NYC.

Consistent with the community-based participatory research values of our overall Safe and Just Cleaners Study and following the model of Public Health 3.0, we were committed as a community–academic partnership to using our data to influence policy to improve workers' social and economic conditions. Our community partner, Make the Road New York, is a major immigrant advocacy organization in New York, and it responded to these findings by providing essential emergency support through food pantries and financial assistance. Beyond these stopgap measures, it prioritized promoting policies to improve financial equity. Make the Road New York, in coalition with other community organizations and supported by data from our study, successfully advocated New York State's appropriation of $2.1 billion for economic support for undocumented immigrant workers excluded from other COVID-19 subsidy programs.[31]

Similarly, the #CancelRent campaign resulted in the passage of the Emergency Rental Assistance Program to prohibit evictions and provide rent subsidies to workers who lost their jobs.[32] Our findings were also used to support advocacy for Coverage for All, a proposed New York State program to provide undocumented immigrants access to affordable health care insurance,[33] although this bill has not yet passed in the New York State legislature as of the publication of this article. Safe and Just Cleaners study participants provided public testimony and joined collective actions to support these campaigns, and many eventually received financial support.

Limitations

Our study was limited to a single major metropolitan area and may not be representative of other populations of housecleaners, although our findings are consistent with other national studies. Our baseline survey was conducted in person and our COVID-19 follow-up survey was administered by telephone, and this may have biased our estimates of the change in our measures of mental and self-rated health, although research suggests that administration methods may not significantly affect responses.[34]

Only a subsample of the population completed the home antibody test kits, and although their self-reported COVID-19 status was similar, their findings may not reflect the entire sample. Also, some of the misclassification between the COVID-19 self-reports and antibody levels may result from antibody levels waning over time or unrecognized asymptomatic participants generating antibodies. Nonetheless, the overall serology findings confirm the high level of COVID-19 infections in our study population.

Of the housecleaners who completed our prepandemic survey, 26% did not participate in this COVID-19 study, and this could introduce some selection bias. Finally, our relatively small study sample size limited the precision of our model estimates and our ability to fully explore the intertwined relationship between COVID-19 infection rates and SBE impacts.

Public Health Implications

Documenting the pandemic's SBE effects illustrates the virtually nonexistent safety net for housecleaners and likely other low-income immigrant workers. Future disease outbreak planning for populations facing disproportionate risks should require, at a minimum, inclusive stopgap measures to mitigate economic insecurity and its sequelae. Broader rethinking of multisectoral social supports that include workers like this study's housecleaners and other immigrant workers would better address workers' and societal health overall. As Park and Chokshi recently wrote, we need to consider "not what social minimum immigrants are owed, but rather how to properly distribute the fundamental benefits and burdens of social cooperation."[35(p3)] AJPH

ABOUT THE AUTHORS

Sherry Baron, Isabel Cuervo, and Dhwanil Shah are with the Barry Commoner Center for Health and the Environment, Queens College, City University of New York, Queens. Ana Gonzalez, and Deysi Flores are with Make the Road New York, Brooklyn, NY. Homero Harari is with the Selikoff Centers for Occupational Health and Institute for Exposomic Research, Icahn School of Medicine at Mount Sinai, New York, NY.

CORRESPONDENCE

Correspondence should be sent to Sherry Baron, Barry Commoner Center for Health and the Environment, Queens College, Remsen 311, 65-30 Kissena Blvd, Flushing, NY 11367 (e-mail: Sherry.Baron@qc.cuny.edu). Reprints can be ordered at http://www.ajph.org by clicking the "Reprints" link.

PUBLICATION INFORMATION

Full Citation: Baron S, Cuervo I, Shah D, Gonzalez A, Harari H, Flores D. COVID-19 infections, pandemic-related social and economic impacts, and changes to mental and self-rated health among Latinx immigrant housecleaners in New York City: the Safe and Just Cleaners Study. *Am J Public Health*. 2023;113(8):893–903.

Acceptance Date: April 18, 2023.

DOI: https://doi.org/10.2105/AJPH.2023.307324

CONTRIBUTORS

S. Baron led, and I. Cuervo and D. Flores assisted with, study design conceptualization, data collection supervision, and statistical analysis. D. Shah analyzed the data. A. Gonzalez led the data collection. A. Gonzalez and H. Harari assisted with study design. D. Flores was the principal contact with the project community partner, Make the Road New York. All authors drafted and revised the article and approved the final version.

ACKNOWLEDGMENTS

Support for this research was provided by the National Institute of Environmental Health Sciences, National Institutes of Health (grant NIEHS 1R01ES027890).

We would like to acknowledge the time, energy, and commitment of all the housecleaners who participated in this study. Maria Baldwin provided support with REDCap programming. The following individuals provided support with development and administration of the survey or survey materials: Flaviana Linares, Lilia Osorio, Jasmine Olivera, Yazmin Gonzalez, Martha Carballo, Rocío Lopez, Janet Rolón Frye, María Lopez, Kelly Martinez, Ana Restrepo, and Madelin Baez. Anonymous peer reviewers provided helpful input during the review process.

Note: The content is solely the responsibility of the authors and does not necessarily represent the official views of the NIH.

CONFLICTS OF INTERESTS

The authors have no conflicts of interests to declare.

HUMAN PARTICIPANT PROTECTION

The City University of New York institutional review board approved this study (protocol 2016-1506-QC).

REFERENCES

1. Mackey K, Ayers CK, Kondo KK, et al. Racial and ethnic disparities in COVID-19–related infections, hospitalizations, and deaths: a systematic review. *Ann Intern Med*. 2021;174(3):362–373. https://doi.org/10.7326/M20-6306

2. Đoàn LN, Chong SK, Misra S, Kwon SC, Yi SS. Immigrant communities and COVID-19: strengthening the public health response. *Am J Public Health.* 2021;111(suppl 3):S224–S231. https://doi.org/10.2105/AJPH.2021.306433
3. DeSalvo KB, Kadakia KT. Public Health 3.0 after COVID-19-reboot or upgrade? *Am J Public Health.* 2021;111(suppl 3):S179–S181. https://doi.org/10.2105/AJPH.2021.306501
4. Riley WT, Borja SE, Hooper MW, et al. National Institutes of Health social and behavioral research in response to the SARS-CoV2 pandemic. *Transl Behav Med.* 2020;10(4):857–861. https://doi.org/10.1093/tbm/ibaa075
5. Baron S, Cuervo I, Winkel G, Flores D, Gonzalez A, Harari H. Employment quality and mental and self-reported health inequities among Latinx housecleaners: the Safe and Just Cleaners Study. *Int J Environ Res Public Health.* 2022;19(23):15973. https://doi.org/10.3390/ijerph192315973
6. Hall M, Greenman E. The occupational cost of being illegal in the United States: legal status, job hazards, and compensating differentials. *Int Migr Rev.* 2015;49(2):406–442. https://doi.org/10.1111/imre.12090
7. Wolfe J, Kandra J, Engdahl L, Shierholz H. Domestic workers chartbook. May 14, 2020. Available at: https://files.epi.org/pdf/194214.pdf. Accessed January 26, 2023.
8. Harris PA, Taylor R, Minor BL, et al. The REDCap consortium: building an international community of software platform partners. *J Biomed Inform.* 2019;95:103208. https://doi.org/10.1016/j.jbi.2019.103208
9. Lieberman-Cribbin W, Tuminello S, Flores RM, Taioli E. Disparities in COVID-19 testing and positivity in New York City. *Am J Prev Med.* 2020;59(3):326–332. https://doi.org/10.1016/j.amepre.2020.06.005
10. Hamilton CM, Strader LC, Pratt JG, et al. The PhenX toolkit: get the most from your measures. *Am J Epidemiol.* 2011;174(3):253–260. https://doi.org/10.1093/aje/kwr193
11. Gundersen C, Engelhard EE, Crumbaugh AS, Seligman HK. Brief assessment of food insecurity accurately identifies high-risk US adults. *Public Health Nutr.* 2017;20(8):1367–1371. https://doi.org/10.1017/S1368980017000180
12. Radloff LS. The CES-D scale: a self-report depression scale for research in the general population. *Appl Psychol Meas.* 1977;1(3):385–401. https://doi.org/10.1177/014662167700100306
13. Cohen S, Kamarck T, Mermelstein R. A global measure of perceived stress. *J Health Soc Behav.* 1983;24(4):385–396. https://doi.org/10.2307/2136404
14. Idler EL, Benyamini Y. Self-rated health and mortality: a review of twenty-seven community studies. *J Health Soc Behav.* 1997;38(1):21–37. https://doi.org/10.2307/2955359
15. Perera MJ, Brintz CE, Birnbaum-Weitzman O, et al. Factor structure of the Perceived Stress Scale-10 (PSS) across English and Spanish language responders in the HCHS/SOL Sociocultural Ancillary Study. *Psychol Assess.* 2017;29(3):320–328. https://doi.org/10.1037/pas0000336
16. Sullivan PS, Sailey C, Guest JL, et al. Detection of SARS-CoV-2 RNA and antibodies in diverse samples: protocol to validate the sufficiency of provider-observed, home-collected blood, saliva, and oropharyngeal samples. *JMIR Public Health Surveill.* 2020;6(2):e19054. https://doi.org/10.2196/19054
17. Hall EW, Luisi N, Zlotorzynska M, et al. Willingness to use home collection methods to provide specimens for SARS-CoV-2/COVID-19 research: survey study. *J Med Internet Res.* 2020;22(9):e19471. https://doi.org/10.2196/19471
18. Siegler AJ, Sullivan PS, Sanchez T, et al. Protocol for a national probability survey using home specimen collection methods to assess prevalence and incidence of SARS-CoV-2 infection and antibody response. *Ann Epidemiol.* 2020;49:50–60. https://doi.org/10.1016/j.annepidem.2020.07.015
19. Andresen EM, Malmgren JA, Carter WB, Patrick DL. Screening for depression in well older adults: evaluation of a short form of the CES-D. *Am J Prev Med.* 1994;10(2):77–84. https://doi.org/10.1016/S0749-3797(18)30622-6
20. MDApp. Perceived Stress Scale (PSS) calculator. Available at: https://www.mdapp.co/perceived-stress-scale-pss-calculator-389. Accessed January 25, 2023.
21. New York City Health. COVID-19: data. Trends and totals. Available at: https://www1.nyc.gov/site/doh/covid/covid-19-data-totals.page. Accessed January 25, 2023.
22. Jones JM, Stone M, Sulaeman H, et al. Estimated US infection- and vaccine-induced SARS-CoV-2 seroprevalence based on blood donations, July 2020–May 2021. *JAMA.* 2021;326(14):1400–1409. https://doi.org/10.1001/jama.2021.15161
23. Vindegaard N, Benros ME. COVID-19 pandemic and mental health consequences: systematic review of the current evidence. *Brain Behav Immun.* 2020;89:531–542. https://doi.org/10.1016/j.bbi.2020.05.048
24. McFadden SM, Demeke J, Dada D, et al. Confidence and hesitancy during the early roll-out of COVID-19 vaccines among Black, Hispanic, and undocumented immigrant communities: a review. *J Urban Health.* 2022;99(1):3–14. https://doi.org/10.1007/s11524-021-00588-1
25. Strassle PD, Stewart AL, Quintero SM, et al. COVID-19–related discrimination among racial/ethnic minorities and other marginalized communities in the United States. *Am J Public Health.* 2022;112(3):453–466. https://doi.org/10.2105/AJPH.2021.306594
26. Lauren BN, Silver ER, Faye AS, et al. Predictors of households at risk for food insecurity in the United States during the COVID-19 pandemic. *Public Health Nutr.* 2021;24(12):3929–3936. https://doi.org/10.1017/S136898002100035
27. Linton SL, Leifheit KM, McGinty EE, Barry CL, Pollack CE. Association between housing insecurity, psychological distress, and self-rated health among US adults during the COVID-19 pandemic. *JAMA Netw Open.* 2021;4(9):e2127772. https://doi.org/10.1001/jamanetworkopen.2021.27772
28. Kourti A, Stavridou A, Panagouli E, et al. Domestic violence during the COVID-19 pandemic: a systematic review. *Trauma Violence Abuse.* 2023;24(2):719–745. https://doi.org/10.1177/15248380211038690
29. Evans ML, Lindauer M, Farrell ME. A pandemic within a pandemic—intimate partner violence during COVID-19. *N Engl J Med.* 2020;383(24):2302–2304. https://doi.org/10.1056/NEJMp2024046
30. National Domestic Workers Alliance. 6 months in crisis: the impact of COVID-19 on domestic workers. October 1, 2020. Available at: https://www.domesticworkers.org/reports-and-publications/6-months-in-crisis-the-impact-of-covid-19-on-domestic-workers. Accessed January 24, 2022.
31. New York State Department of Labor. Excluded workers fund. November 2021. Available at: https://dol.ny.gov/system/files/documents/2022/01/nys-ewf-whitepaper-november21_01-26-22_0.pdf. Accessed January 17, 2023.
32. New York State Office of Temporary and Disability Assistance. Emergency rental assistance program. Available at: https://otda.ny.gov/programs/emergency-rental-assistance/#overview. Accessed January 25, 2023.
33. Lander B. Economic benefits of coverage for all. March 15, 2022. Available at: https://comptroller.nyc.gov/reports/economic-benefits-of-coverage-for-all. Accessed January 17, 2023.
34. Aneshensel CS, Frerichs RR, Clark VA, Yokopenic PA. Measuring depression in the community: a comparison of telephone and personal interviews. *Public Opin Q.* 1982;46(1):110–121. https://doi.org/10.1086/268703
35. Park JK, Chokshi DA. Toward a new standard of health for immigrants in the United States. *Lancet Reg Health Am.* 2022;10:100238. https://doi.org/10.1016/j.lana.2022.100238

SARS-CoV-2 Cases Reported on International Arriving and Domestic Flights: United States, January 2020–December 2021

Leigh Ellyn Preston, DrPH, Araceli Rey, MPH, Simone Dumas, MPH, Andrea Rodriguez, MPH, Alida M. Gertz, MD, Kristin C. Delea, MPH, Francisco Alvarado-Ramy, MD, Deborah L. Christensen, PhD, Clive Brown, MBBS, and Tai-Ho Chen, MD

Objectives. To describe trends in the number of air travelers categorized as infectious with SARS-CoV-2 (severe acute respiratory syndrome coronavirus 2; the virus that causes COVID-19) in the context of total US COVID-19 vaccinations administered, and overall case counts of SARS-CoV-2 in the United States.

Methods. We searched the Quarantine Activity Reporting System (QARS) database for travelers with inbound international or domestic air travel, a positive SARS-CoV-2 lab result, and a surveillance categorization of SARS-CoV-2 infection reported during January 2020 to December 2021. Travelers were categorized as infectious during travel if they had arrival dates from 2 days before to 10 days after symptom onset or a positive viral test.

Results. We identified 80 715 persons meeting our inclusion criteria; 67 445 persons (83.6%) had at least 1 symptom reported. Of 67 445 symptomatic passengers, 43 884 (65.1%) reported an initial symptom onset date after their flight arrival date. The number of infectious travelers mirrored the overall number of US SARS-CoV-2 cases.

Conclusions. Most travelers in the study were asymptomatic during travel, and therefore unknowingly traveled while infectious. During periods of high community transmission, it is important for travelers to stay up to date with COVID-19 vaccinations and consider wearing a high-quality mask to decrease the risk of transmission. (*Am J Public Health*. 2023;113(8):904–908. https://doi.org/10.2105/AJPH.2023.307325)

AJPH August 2023, Vol 113, No. 8

Transmission of SARS-CoV-2 (severe acute respiratory syndrome coronavirus 2; the virus that causes COVID-19) has been correlated with travel.[1–3] Previous studies indicated that SARS-CoV-2 transmission events during and after air travel can be reduced with prevention strategies, including masking.[4]

The Centers for Disease Control and Prevention (CDC) operates 20 quarantine stations at US ports of entry with high volumes of arriving international travelers.[5] Quarantine station personnel respond to ill travelers reported during travel and collect information on ill travelers identified after travel is completed. These data are entered and stored in an electronic record-keeping system, the Quarantine Activity Reporting System (QARS).

During the COVID-19 pandemic, partners reported to the CDC persons infected with SARS-CoV-2 with recent travel who were identified during routine case investigations and contact tracing.[6] We performed a retrospective record review to describe the trends and characteristics of travelers identified as infectious with SARS-CoV-2 in the context of the initiation of US COVID-19–associated travel policies, US COVID-19 vaccinations administered, and US SARS-CoV-2 case counts.

METHODS

We queried the QARS database for all travelers with inbound international or domestic air travel with a positive SARS-CoV-2 lab result and a surveillance categorization of SARS-CoV-2 infection reported during January 2020 through December 2021.

We classified cases as infectious during travel if they were reported as having laboratory-confirmed SARS-CoV-2 infection by a viral (i.e., nucleic acid amplification or antigen) test, and met 1 of the following conditions:

- Reported COVID-19–compatible symptoms and flight arrival within the traveler's infectious period, or
- No reported COVID-19–compatible symptoms but flight arrival during the traveler's infectious period.[7]

We determined infectious periods on the basis of CDC quarantine and isolation guidance during this period[7] and defined them for analysis as follows:

- Symptomatic travelers: from 2 days before symptom onset or initial positive viral test, whichever was earlier, until 10 days after.
- Asymptomatic travelers: from 2 days before initial positive viral test until 10 days after.

Travelers with multiple legs of travel could be considered infectious on multiple flights. Although we did not measure infectiousness, we refer to passengers as infectious if they were within the infectious period described in the previous paragraphs.

We documented trends among travelers classified as infectious along with trends in overall traveler volume for domestic and inbound international flights, as well as trends in overall US SARS-CoV-2 cases and vaccination rates. Travel volume on domestic and inbound international flights was provided by the US Customs and Border Protection via the CDC's Division of Global Migration and Quarantine's Office of Innovation Development Evaluation and Analysis. We obtained the overall number of people with COVID-19 in the United States and vaccination information through the CDC's COVID Data Tracker.[8]

We plotted key mitigation policies implemented during our study period to provide context. The CDC issued orders aimed at reducing the number of people infected with SARS-CoV-2 entering the United States. Beginning January 26, 2021, the United States required all passengers arriving from international destinations to show proof of a negative test result for, or documented recovery from, SARS-CoV-2.[9] Beginning February 1, 2021, the CDC required the use of masks on public transportation conveyances, including commercial aircraft, or on the premises of domestic transportation hubs.[10] COVID-19 vaccines were initially made available to persons aged 16 years and older in mid-December 2020.[11]

RESULTS

During January 2020 through December 2021, 80 715 persons infectious with SARS-CoV-2 were reported to the CDC as having traveled on 125 135 domestic and 14 678 international inbound flights. Our data included 38 096 (47.2%) travelers identified as female, 35 186 (43.6%) identified as male, and 7433 (9.2%) reports in which gender was not specified. The mean age of passengers was 38.5 years (median = 36 years; range = 0–102 years).

Of the 80 715 travelers, 8523 (10.6%) were reported to be asymptomatic, 67 445 (83.6%) had at least 1 symptom reported, and 4747 (5.9%) were missing information on symptoms. Of 67 445 symptomatic passengers, 31 155 (46.1%) had onset of at least 1 symptom on or before their flight arrival date, and 43 884 (65.1%) reported an initial symptom onset date after their flight arrival date. These groups are not mutually exclusive, as passengers may have traveled on multiple flights across multiple days.

Trends in the monthly numbers of infectious travelers and of all travelers (regardless of SARS-CoV-2 infection status), vaccinations administered, and new SARS-CoV-2 infections in the United States are shown in Figure 1, along with the timing of key mitigation efforts affecting both domestic travelers and arriving international passengers. Figure 1 also shows new SARS-CoV-2 cases and the number of infectious travelers, along with date of initiation of CDC travel mitigation efforts. During fall 2020, the number of infectious travelers rose along with new US SARS-CoV-2 cases, peaking in January 2021; overall travel volume did not change. After January 2021, the number of infectious travelers fell sharply, as did overall monthly US cases, and then began to increase again as travel volume increased in March and April 2021. After April 2021, the monthly number of infectious travelers diverged from overall travel volume and closely paralleled the number of newly infected persons until July 2021. In July 2021, when overall travel volume peaked, the numbers of infectious travelers and new US cases also rose, peaking in August 2021 (Figure 1).

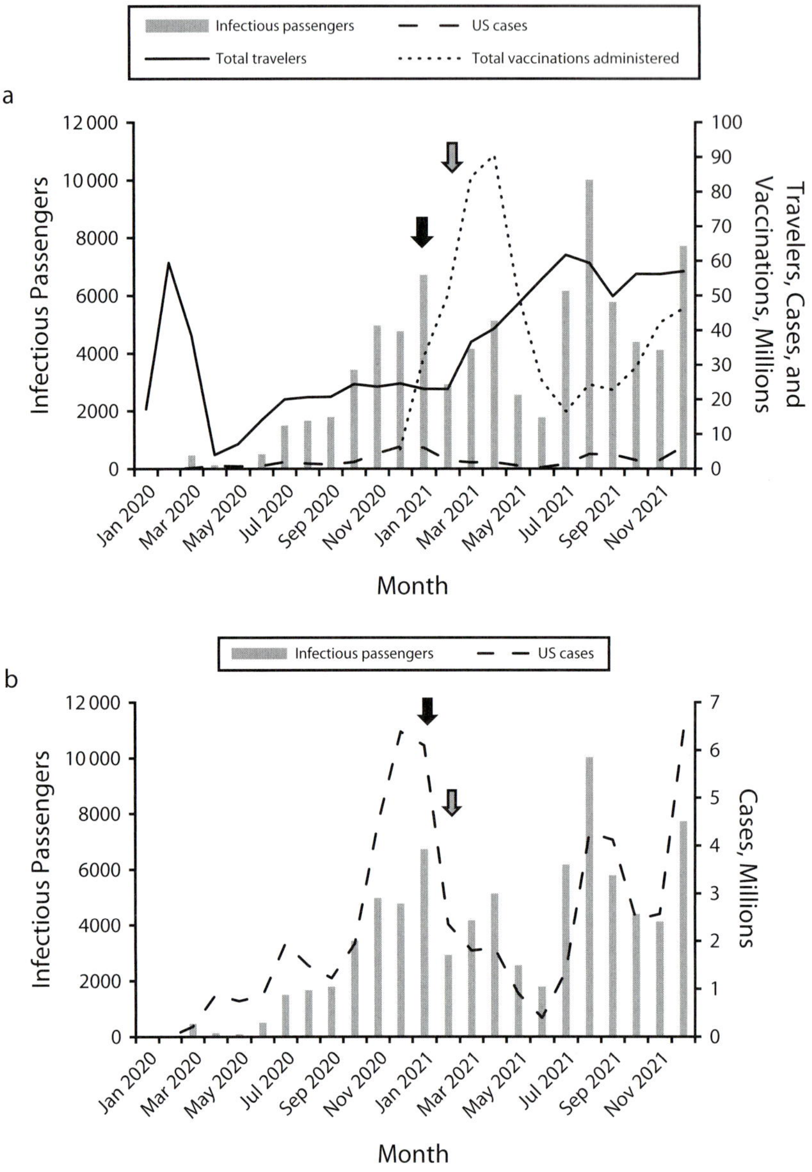

FIGURE 1— Number of Infectious Passengers by (a) Number of US SARS-CoV-2 Cases, Number of Vaccines Administered in the United States, and Overall US Travel Volume per Month; and (b) Number of US SARS-CoV-2 Cases per Month: January 2020–December 2021

Note. SARS-CoV-2 (severe acute respiratory syndrome coronavirus 2) is the virus that causes COVID-19. Travel volume was determined by international inbound and domestic flights. Black arrow indicates the month when the Centers for Disease Control and Prevention (CDC) initiated testing requirements upon entry to the United States (January 26, 2021) and gray arrow indicates the date the CDC mandated face masks on public transport in the United States (February 1, 2021).

In early 2021, the CDC issued orders aimed at reducing the number of people infected with SARS-CoV-2 entering the United States, indicated in Figure 1 by black and gray arrows.[9,10] A substantial drop in the numbers of infectious travelers and US cases can be seen in the months following these orders, concurrent with increased vaccinations administered, but numbers of infectious travelers and new SARS-CoV-2 cases rebounded during the summer months of 2021, following the overall trend in the number of travelers (Figure 1). This could be attributable to the increased number of US cases attributed to the Delta variant.

DISCUSSION

In general, beginning in the summer of 2020, the trend in the monthly number of infectious travelers follows the trend in new US SARS-CoV-2 cases. The decline in both infectious passengers and US cases in early 2021 could be attributable to several factors, including vaccine uptake, decreased community transmission, and unmeasured mitigation efforts. It is difficult to measure the direct impact of the CDC travel mitigation efforts on the number of infectious travelers because of the indirect way in which data were collected regarding adherence to the testing and masking requirements and other complex factors that affect transmission.

Of 67 445 symptomatic infectious passengers, 63% reported a symptom onset date after their flight arrival date. This indicates the potential for precautionary steps, including mask use and vaccination, to prevent transmission of infectious diseases—including asymptomatic transmission—during travel.

Our data likely underestimate the true number of persons who traveled while infectious, as persons who were infectious with SARS-CoV-2 during travel may not have been reported to the CDC. As community spread of SARS-CoV-2 increased, state and local health department partners prioritized other activities over case reporting to maximize their public health impact. Additionally, persons infected with SARS-CoV-2 may not have reported travel to public health to avoid cancelling their travel. These infected persons would not be captured in our data set.

The strengths of this analysis included a large data set; however, it is unclear whether it is representative of the population of US residents who travel. Because our data set was restricted to travelers with proof of laboratory confirmation in the report, all cases documented in our analysis were positive for SARS-CoV-2 by viral test. Travelers who were ill but not tested for SARS-CoV-2 would not be captured.

PUBLIC HEALTH IMPLICATIONS

The number of infectious travelers mirrored the overall number of US SARS-CoV-2 cases. Fewer than half of the travelers classified as infectious during their flight were symptomatic during travel; therefore, some travelers unknowingly travel while infectious. It is important for travelers to stay current on COVID-19 vaccinations to decrease the risk of severe disease and consider wearing a high-quality mask during air travel, particularly travelers at higher risk of severe disease and when community transmission is high. AJPH

ABOUT THE AUTHORS

Leigh Ellyn Preston, Araceli Rey, Simone Dumas, Andrea Rodriguez, Alida Gertz, Kristin C. Delea, Francisco Alvarado-Ramy, Deborah L. Christensen, Clive Brown, and Tai-Ho Chen are with the CDC COVID-19 Ports of Entry Team, Atlanta, GA.

CORRESPONDENCE

Correspondence should be sent to Leigh Ellyn Preston, 1600 Clifton Rd, Atlanta, GA 30324 (e-mail: lpreston@cdc.gov). Reprints can be ordered at http://www.ajph.org by clicking the "Reprints" link.

PUBLICATION INFORMATION

Full Citation: Preston LE, Rey A, Dumas S, et al. SARS-CoV-2 cases reported on international arriving and domestic flights: United States, January 2020–December 2021. *Am J Public Health*. 2023;113(8):904–908.

Acceptance Date: April 18, 2023.

DOI: https://doi.org/10.2105/AJPH.2023.307325

CONTRIBUTORS

L. E. Preston performed data cleaning, data analysis, and manuscript writing and editing. A. Rey performed data analysis and manuscript writing and editing. S. Dumas and A. Rodriguez performed data cleaning and manuscript editing. A. M. Gertz and T.-H. Chen performed manuscript writing and editing. K. C. Delea, F. Alvarado-Ramy, D. L. Christensen, and C. Brown performed manuscript editing.

ACKNOWLEDGMENTS

This project was supported in part by an appointment to the Research Participation Program at the Centers for Disease Control and Prevention (CDC) administered by the Oak Ridge Institute for Science and Education through an interagency agreement between the US Department of Energy and the CDC.

We acknowledge and thank all the operational staff and deployers at the CDC quarantine stations.

Note. The findings and conclusions in this report are those of the authors and do not necessarily represent the official position of the Centers for Disease Control and Prevention.

CONFLICTS OF INTEREST

The authors have no conflicts of interest to disclose.

HUMAN PARTICIPANT PROTECTION

Data analyzed and presented in this report were deemed part of routine surveillance operations and granted a non-research determination in CDC review.

REFERENCES

1. Kraemer MU, Yang CH, Gutierrez B, et al. The effect of human mobility and control measures on the COVID-19 epidemic in China. *Science*. 2020;368(6490):493–497. https://doi.org/10.1126/science.abb4218
2. Li Y, Hou S, Zhang Y, et al. Effect of travel restrictions of Wuhan city against COVID-19: a modified SEIR model analysis. *Disaster Med Public Health Prep*. 2022;16(4):1431–1437. https://doi.org/10.1017/dmp.2021.5
3. Fareed Z, Ghaemi Asl M, Irfan M, et al. Exploring the co-movements between COVID-19 pandemic and international air traffic: a global perspective based on wavelet analysis. *Int Migr*. 2022;Epub ahead of print June 9, 2022. https://doi.org/10.1111/imig.13026
4. Zhang J, Qin F, Qin X, et al. Transmission of SARS-CoV-2 during air travel: a descriptive and modelling study. *Ann Med*. 2021;53(1):1569–1575. https://doi.org/10.1080/07853890.2021.1973084
5. Centers for Disease Control and Prevention. US quarantine stations. Available at: https://www.cdc.gov/quarantine/quarantine-stations-us.html. Accessed September 15, 2022.

6. Centers for Disease Control and Prevention. Protecting travelers' health from airport to community: investigation contagious diseases on flights. Available at: https://www.cdc.gov/quarantine/contact-investigation.html. Accessed September 12, 2022.
7. Centers for Disease Control and Prevention. Isolation and precautions for people with COVID-19. Available at: https://www.cdc.gov/coronavirus/2019-ncov/your-health/isolation.html?CDC_AA_refVal=https%3A%2F%2Fwww.cdc.gov%2Fcoronavirus%2F2019-ncov%2Fyour-health%2Fquarantine-isolation.html. Accessed September 12, 2022.
8. Centers for Disease Control and Prevention. COVID Data Tracker. Available at: https://covid.cdc.gov/covid-data-tracker/#datatracker-home. Accessed September 12, 2022.
9. Centers for Disease Control and Prevention. Requirement for negative pre-departure COVID-19 test result or documentation of recovery from COVID-19 for all airline or other aircraft passengers arriving into the United States from any foreign country: archive. Available at: https://www.cdc.gov/quarantine/fr-proof-negative-test.html. Accessed September 15, 2022.
10. Centers for Disease Control and Prevention. Order: wearing of face masks while on conveyances and at transportation hubs. Available at: https://www.cdc.gov/quarantine/masks/mask-travel-guidance.html. Accessed September 15, 2022.
11. Oliver S, Gargano J, Marin M, et al. The Advisory Committee on Immunization Practices' interim recommendation for use of Pfizer-BioNTech COVID-19 vaccine—United States, December 2020. *MMWR Morb Mortal Wkly Rep.* 2020;69:1922–1924. http://dx.doi.org/10.15585/mmwr.mm6950e2

Promising Practices Observed in High-Throughput COVID-19 Vaccination Sites in the United States, February–May 2021

Caitlin E. McColloch, MDP, Marsha E. Samson, PhD, MPH, MSHSA, KaeAnne Parris, MPH, Amy Stewart, MPH, Judith A. Robinson, JD, MPH, MIS, Barbara Cooper, MSPH, Eboni Galloway, PhD, MPH, Robert Garcia, MSW, MPH, Zunera Gilani, PhD, MPH, Bina Jayapaul-Philip, PhD, Paul Lucas, MS, Kimberly H. Nguyen, DrPH, MS, Rebecca S. Noe, MN, MPH, FNP-BC, Aimée-Rika T. Trudeau, MPH, and Erin D. Kennedy, DVM, MS, MPH

See also Brandt, p. 836.

Objectives. To identify promising practices for implementing COVID-19 vaccination sites.

Methods. The Centers for Disease Control and Prevention (CDC) and Federal Emergency Management Agency (FEMA) assessed high-throughput COVID-19 vaccination sites across the United States, including Puerto Rico, after COVID-19 vaccinations began. Site assessors conducted site observations and interviews with site staff. Qualitative data were compiled and thematically analyzed.

Results. CDC and FEMA conducted 134 assessments of high-throughput vaccination sites in 25 states and Puerto Rico from February 12 to May 28, 2021. Promising practices were identified across facility, clinical, and cross-cutting operational areas and related to 6 main themes: addressing health equity, leveraging partnerships, optimizing site design and flow, communicating through visual cues, using quick response codes, and prioritizing risk management and quality control.

Conclusions. These practices might help planning and implementation of future vaccination operations for COVID-19, influenza, and other vaccine-preventable diseases.

Public Health Implications. These practices can be considered by vaccination planners and providers to strengthen their vaccination site plans and implementation of future high-throughput vaccination sites. (*Am J Public Health*. 2023;113(8):909–918. https://doi.org/10.2105/AJPH.2023.307331)

AJPH August 2023, Vol 113, No. 8

As COVID-19 vaccine development was under way in 2020, public health agencies and health care providers across the United States prepared to administer COVID-19 vaccinations on a large scale.[1] Although certain providers had previous experience with large-scale vaccination campaigns, such as for the 2009 H1N1 pandemic, many had limited experience providing vaccinations at the unprecedented scale and urgency of the COVID-19 pandemic or managing the demanding and differing COVID-19 vaccine storage and handling requirements.[2] Providers including, but not limited to, health departments, pharmacies, and community health centers had to quickly determine how to best implement and manage COVID-19 vaccination sites in their communities.

The Centers for Disease Control and Prevention (CDC) partnered with the 64 federally funded state, local, and territorial health department immunization programs (hereafter called immunization programs) to plan for the rapid administration of COVID-19 vaccines. Immunization programs received COVID-19 vaccines and vaccine-related funds according to each program's distribution plan.[1,3] These plans included how and where immunization programs would distribute federally supplied vaccines to providers that managed COVID-19 vaccination sites in their jurisdictions. A core strategy of the distribution plans included implementation of high-throughput vaccination sites, sometimes referred to as mass vaccination sites, used to vaccinate many persons rapidly and efficiently. Sites included fixed facility, drive-through, and mobile sites, and were established in different settings such as pharmacies, sports arenas, and universities.[4] The Federal Emergency Management Agency (FEMA) also partnered with immunization programs to establish and support high-throughput sites called community vaccination centers (CVCs).[5]

To become an authorized vaccination provider and receive vaccine, providers were required to enroll in CDC's COVID-19 Vaccination Program and agree to manage, store, and administer vaccines in accordance with all federal and manufacturer guidelines.[6] Guidelines were associated with cold-chain management, vaccine preparation and administration, billing, and reporting. Immunization programs and providers received guidance documents and training materials developed by the federal government and their partners outlining COVID-19–specific procedures, including for implementing high-throughput sites, based on previous pandemic response and immunization guidance.[3,5,7–10]

To understand how providers at high-throughput COVID-19 vaccination sites implemented the guidance, CDC and FEMA conducted site assessments during the beginning of high-throughput COVID-19 vaccinations in the United States. Another objective of these assessments was to capture promising practices to share with current and future providers operating these or similar types of sites in the future. We evaluated data gathered by CDC and FEMA from more than 100 sites across the United States to identify promising practices for implementing high-throughput vaccination.

METHODS

We describe the FEMA- and CDC-led vaccination site assessment methods here.

FEMA-Led Vaccination Site Assessments

FEMA's Continuous Improvement Program initiated CVC site visits in February 2021. Initially, Continuous Improvement Program teams were composed of staff from FEMA, CDC, the Department of Defense, and US Department of Health and Human Services (HHS), who had expertise in different aspects of high-throughput vaccination. When the initial sites were opened, given limited federal staff because of the scope of nationwide operations, FEMA deployed 1 or 2 staff with emergency management expertise to a site for 1 or 2 weeks to capture lessons learned for future site openings. By the end of March, FEMA shifted its deployment model for assessments to a rotating basis for 1 or 2 days, every 2 to 3 weeks. This model was staffed by 3 or 4 staff representing emergency management, medical, and public health backgrounds.

Continuous Improvement Program teams assessed best practices, concerns, and lessons learned for implementing CVC sites across the topics of facility operations, safety, staffing, vaccine recipient experience, facility support, community outreach, and clinical operations. Observations were collated into a report at the end of each visit; FEMA summarized individual site reports into a combined report.

CDC-Led Vaccination Site Assessments

In March 2021, CDC began recruiting immunization programs to participate in CDC's COVID-19 vaccination site assessment project. First, COVID-19 sites across the United States and the territory of Puerto Rico with the highest proportion of doses received were identified using vaccine distribution data.[11] Immunization programs were recruited based on existence of vaccination sites in their jurisdictions that made up the highest proportion of doses received and accounting for geographic diversity across all HHS regions (≥ 1 immunization program per region). Next, specific sites were selected in consultation with immunization programs to include sites responsible for a substantial proportion of vaccinations administered and to align with the immunization program's assessment goals, such as inclusion of sites not yet visited by the immunization program and sites managed by new partners. CVC sites were excluded. CDC sent teams of at least 2 assessors to each site to observe operations and interview staff; assessments typically lasted 2 to 4 hours.

CDC assessment teams used a data collection tool based on 4 elements: billing and documentation, storage and handling, vaccination procedures, and ancillary supply kits. Subject matter experts at CDC developed and piloted the tool, which was derived from a questionnaire used to assess Vaccines for Children program providers.[12] The tool included a section to capture data regarding the site visit setting and a notes section to capture promising practices. A promising practice was any approach to organize or implement a COVID-19 vaccination site that was observed to have a positive effect on efficiency or ability to adhere to all federal and manufacturer guidelines. Teams were instructed to capture these data through observation and interviews with site staff and enter data into a database after each site visit.

Coding Process and Data Analysis

Promising practices were abstracted from the CDC database and FEMA reports and organized into a spreadsheet for analysis. Practices that did not comply with immunization best practices were excluded. We used an iterative thematic analysis process that included a combination of deductive and inductive coding techniques to organize data and identify themes.[13] An initial list of codes was generated based on sections of CDC's data collection tool and FEMA summary reports. Then, 2 analysts independently coded 20% of the data to revise codes and develop the initial codebook. Analysts compared coded segments, discussed discrepancies, and refined the codebook until intercoder reliability reached 80%, at which point the analysts independently coded the remaining data set. Analysts then summarized practices and reviewed patterns within codes to identify themes.

Compiling practices was an iterative process. Given that guidelines for COVID-19 vaccination evolved after data collection and site assessors had various expertise in immunization services, coauthors reviewed the summarized promising practices to identify the most relevant (i.e., important to future COVID-19 high-throughput sites), novel (i.e., unique), and generalizable (i.e., applicable in different settings) based on their subject matter expertise (e.g., immunization services, public health preparedness, emergency response). Coauthors scored practices on a scale from 1 to 5, where 1 was the lowest, for each classification (i.e., relevancy, novelty, and generalizability). Then, the group met to select practices to disseminate based on their scores. The list of example practices for dissemination was further refined after input from additional CDC subject matter experts.

We categorized sites that underwent CDC-led assessments based on site setting. The settings included traditional (i.e., pharmacy, health care provider office, health center, medical practice, outpatient clinic, urgent care facility, and public health clinic), nontraditional (i.e., community center, college, technical school, university, temporary or off-site vaccination clinic, point of dispensing, temporary location, mobile clinic, inpatient facility, and workplace), and other or unknown (i.e., the setting was unclear or > 1 setting type was listed). Because we did not have FEMA CVC site setting data, we retrospectively categorized FEMA sites based on the site's name. For example, if the name was a sports arena, we categorized it as nontraditional. We performed descriptive analyses of these data. Although data from CDC-led and FEMA-led assessments did not systematically include information regarding site modality (i.e., walk-through, drive-through, or mobile sites), we looked for and categorized descriptions of site modality in the promising practices data during qualitative analysis.

RESULTS

CDC and FEMA assessors conducted site visits in 134 high-throughput COVID-19 vaccination sites and CVCs across 30 immunization programs in 25 state health departments, 4 city health departments, and 1 territorial health department from February 12 to May 28, 2021 (Figure 1). Most sites were at nontraditional settings (63%; n = 84; Table 1). Of the 96 (72%) CDC-led assessments, 58% (n = 56) were at nontraditional settings. Of the 38 (28%) FEMA-led assessments, 74% (n = 28) were at nontraditional settings.

The final set of codes for the qualitative analysis of promising practice data were organized by facility operations, clinical operations, and cross-cutting codes (Box 1). We identified a range of promising practices across all codes. Table A (available as a supplement to the online version of this article at https://ajph.org) provides a list of examples of promising practices organized by code that subject matter experts considered potentially useful to current or future vaccination providers. Here we highlight 6 overarching themes identified during the thematic analysis process and provide specific examples of a promising practice for each theme (Box 2):

1. Addressing health equity,
2. Leveraging partnerships,
3. Optimizing space and flow,
4. Communicating through visual cues,
5. Using quick response codes, and
6. Prioritizing risk management and quality control.

Addressing Health Equity

The health equity theme is associated with providing equitable access to vaccines and vaccine information regardless of demographics, language, disability status, and other characteristics associated with health disparities (e.g., socioeconomic factors).[14] For example, staff at the site entrance might

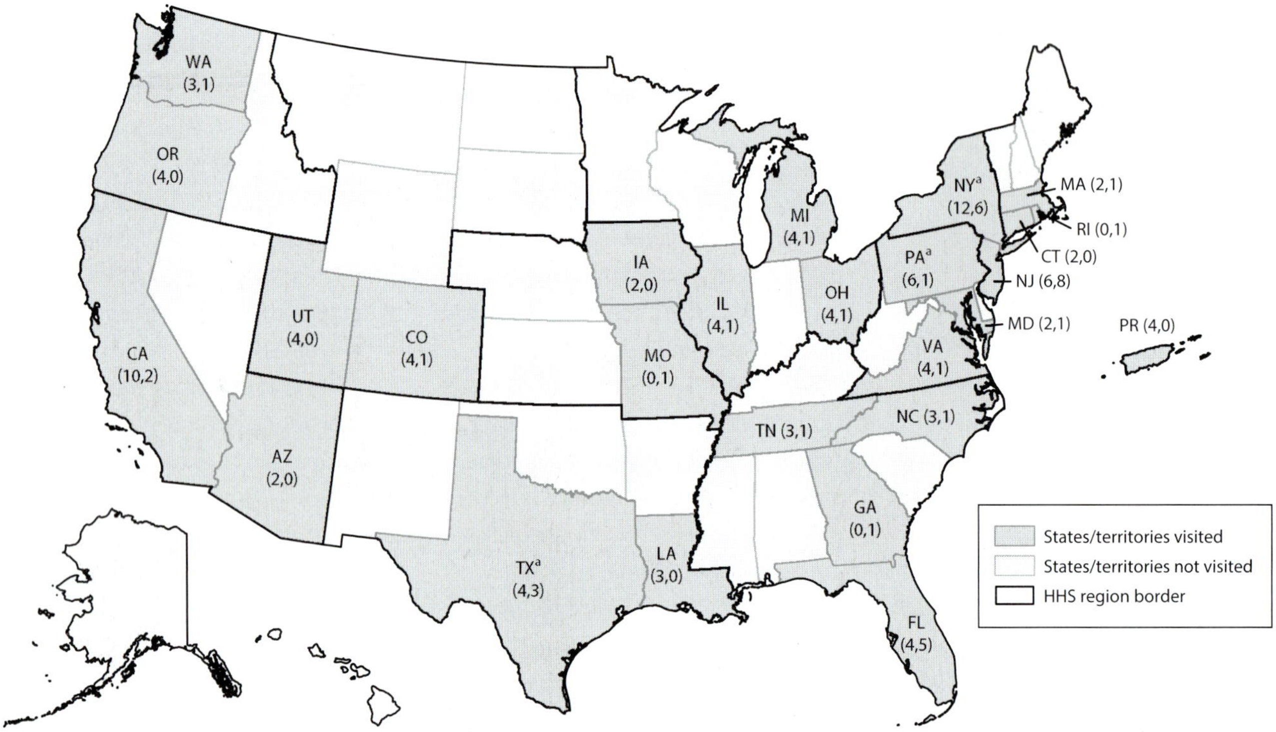

FIGURE 1— Location of State, Local, and Territorial Immunization Programs That Participated in the Centers for Disease Control and Prevention (CDC) and Federal Emergency Management Agency (FEMA) COVID-19 Vaccination Site Assessment Projects Across US Department of Health and Human Services (HHS) Regions: United States, February–May 2021

Note. The number of COVID-19 vaccination sites visited per immunization program jurisdiction is indicated in parentheses with the number of sites visited by CDC followed by the number of sites visited by FEMA.
[a]Includes city immunization programs (New York, NY [4], Philadelphia, PA [2], San Antonio, TX [1], and Houston, TX [1]).

have a language handout to help identify the recipient's language and direct them to appropriate language services, or wheelchair escorts might be available to transport persons with access and functional needs from site entry through the vaccination process. Certain practices included a designated area to accommodate individuals with developmental or emotional access and functional needs that might require privacy or expedited services.

Some site managers collected and tracked data related to race, ethnicity, disability status, language preferences, or transportation barriers at registration to prioritize and refine outreach, such as where to deploy mobile sites or

TABLE 1— Centers for Disease Control and Prevention (CDC)– and Federal Emergency Management Agency (FEMA)–led COVID-19 Vaccination Site Assessments by Setting Type: United States, February 12–May 28, 2021

	Traditional, No. (% of Row)	Nontraditional, No. (% of Row)	Other or Unknown, No. (% of Row)	Total, No. (% of Row)
CDC-led total	26 (27)	56 (58)	14 (15)	96 (100)
FEMA-led total	0 (0)	28 (74)	10 (26)	38 (100)
Total	26 (19)	84 (63)	24 (18)	134 (100)

Note. Setting types include traditional (i.e., pharmacy, health care provider office, health center, medical practice, outpatient clinic, public health clinic, urgent care facility), nontraditional (i.e., community center, college, technical school, university, temporary or off-site vaccination clinic, point of dispensing, temporary location, mobile clinic, inpatient facility, workplace), and other or unknown (i.e., the setting was unclear or > 1 setting was listed).

BOX 1— COVID-19 Vaccination Site Promising Practices Codebook, Centers for Disease Control and Prevention and Federal Emergency Management Agency Site Assessments of COVID-19 Mass Vaccination Sites Across the United States and Puerto Rico: February–May 2021

Operational Area Category	Operational Area Code	Definition (Refers to)
Facility operations	Site management	Site administration, communication, and leadership systems and processes
	Staffing and training	Recruiting and training of staff and volunteers and designating them for certain roles and responsibilities
	Site safety and security	Mitigating hazards and threats (potential or existing) at the site
	Registration and scheduling	Anything related to, or that occurs at or during, appointment registration, scheduling, or check-in
	Outreach	Reaching and recruiting vaccine recipients
Clinical operations	Vaccine preparation	The final stage in the cold chain before administration (i.e., labeling, mixing, and drawing vaccine and diluent into syringes for vaccine administration)
	Vaccine administration	Anything that occurs during the administration stage or at the administration station
	Storage and handling	Cold-chain management: storage units, temperature monitoring, inventory, and vaccine transport
	Lot change	Bringing a new batch of vaccine with a different lot number to the floor for administration
	Recipient observation	Monitoring recipients after vaccination
	Vaccine record card	Anything related to the vaccine recipient's vaccine record card, including producing or updating card
Cross-cutting	Visual cues	Highlighting or pointing out information using, for example, colors, symbols or images, or text
	Quick response (QR) codes	The use of QR codes
	Partnerships	Collaboration with partners (private or public, individuals or organizations or agencies)
	Special populations	Accommodations for specific groups of people, such as individuals with disabilities, individuals who speak languages other than English, or critical infrastructure workforce (e.g., vaccinating staff)
	Public education	What and how information (e.g., site policies, vaccine information) is provided to vaccine recipients
	Site layout and design	Site arrangement and use of space
Other		Emerging themes or anything that does not adequately fit in any other code

which language interpreters to have on site.

Leveraging Partnerships

Leveraging partnerships is associated with ways providers used new or existing public or private partnerships to enhance vaccination sites. For example, some providers partnered with public and private entities with expertise in specific operational areas, such as event planning, crowd control, and serving individuals with disabilities, to facilitate effective site design. Providers leveraged national (e.g., AmeriCorps, National Guard, or Veterans Affairs) and local (e.g., health professional schools, community organizations, or the facility in which the site operates for temporary sites) partnerships to recruit site staff and volunteers. Some site managers partnered with community organizations, religious institutions, media outlets, and public transit authorities to support community outreach, particularly for populations who have been historically underserved by health care services and groups with lower vaccination coverage, which was also associated with the first theme.

Optimizing Space and Flow

Optimizing space and flow is associated with methods of site design and organization. For example, next-in-line recipients moved from the regular queue to a position directly next to the vaccination station to help expedite throughput. Separate vaccination areas were implemented to allow complex situations to

BOX 2— Example Promising Practices by Theme Identified During Centers for Disease Control and Prevention and Federal Emergency Management Agency COVID-19 High-Throughput Vaccination Site Assessments: United States, February 12–May 28, 2021

Theme	Example
Addressing health equity	The site is located within a sports arena. Although it serves 1000 vaccine recipients per day, it was designed to serve 3000. Unused vaccination points of dispensing physically distant from those in use are available for special recipients, including those who might be cognitively disabled, vaccine- or needle-apprehensive, or otherwise requiring more reassurance or other measures. This has allowed all recipients to be more easily and safely vaccinated and minimized the transmission of anxiety to nearby recipients.
Leveraging partnerships	One site reported to have contacted local community services, their health department, welfare services, and church groups to support those who are in culturally segregated groups, the unhoused population, and those without access to cell phones and computers. Churches have been fundamental in reaching individuals and reducing misinterpretation of the intent of the sites, calming people, and building confidence.
Optimizing space or flow	The recipient observation area at one site became a choke point. To ensure sustained throughput while maintaining the required 6-foot separation between vaccine recipients, the site added a tent to the end of the vaccination pathway and began directing recipients into each of the 2 observation areas based on observation requirements (i.e., those needing 15 minutes vs 30 minutes). By expanding its observation capacity, the site was able to maintain its high throughput and provide sheltered observation for its recipients while still adhering to physical distancing requirements.
Communicating through visual cues	To decrease foot traffic near motor vehicles and ensure adequate supplies, site personnel at 1 drive-through site used orange traffic safety cones to indicate needed supplies. Staff placed a cone outside the tent facing upright if more vaccine was needed, laid down facing the tent if they were out of vaccine, and laid down facing away from the tent if they needed a 1.5-inch needle.
Using quick response (QR) codes	The site uses QR codes to track vaccine inventory. QR codes linked to the vaccine inventory tracking system are placed on vaccine storage units. When mobile team members pick up vaccine, they scan the QR code and log the amount of vaccine they took. They do the same process to check vaccine back into the storage unit, when appropriate.
Prioritizing risk management and quality control	A few individuals below the allowable age were vaccinated. Therefore, site leadership developed a checklist, which includes instructions for verifying recipient age that must be completed for each recipient before a vaccine syringe is provided to the vaccinator.

be triaged and handled with the appropriate attention without holding up the primary administration queues. Practices in this theme are also associated with placement of staff, such as stationing a clinician at the check-in station to help address any medical questions or concerns among vaccine recipients before they get to the vaccination station. Additional approaches involved the organization of site areas, including delineating space for 15-minute versus 30-minute postvaccination observation times and designating areas for vaccine-specific reconstitution and administration that are only accessible through vaccine-specific entrances.

Communicating Through Visual Cues

The fourth theme is associated with the use of different types of visual cues, such as posters, monitors, stickers, tape, flags, and vests to communicate with the vaccine recipients and site staff and to promote site safety. For vaccine recipients, visual cues communicated site policies (e.g., signage to indicate where to pick up and drop off wheelchairs), recipient support (e.g., availability of on-site translators), wayfinding (e.g., color-coded signage and tape to direct people to queuing lines), and educational information (e.g., monitors located in queuing lines to display slideshows or videos with COVID-19 vaccine facts). Visual cues were also used as staff communication tools—for example, color-coded flags or cones to indicate when supplies or support was needed at a vaccination station, color-coded stickers to identify vaccine recipients at higher risk for adverse events in the observation area, and storage and handling protocol reminders placed in obvious locations on storage units. Visual cues promoted site safety, including color-coded stickers or wristbands to identify staff who have passed daily COVID-19 safety screening.

Using Quick Response Codes

The fifth theme is associated with the use of quick response (QR) codes to share and collect information. Although there were promising practices that related to other digital technology, such as 2-dimensional (2D) barcodes to record vaccine information (e.g., lot number and expiration date), this theme focuses on QR codes because of the frequency of mentions in the data. Providers linked vaccination information to QR codes and displayed the QR codes throughout sites on large posters or adhered to the backs of chairs in the observation area. Sometimes these strategies were used to collect feedback from recipients and linked QR codes to online surveys. QR codes were also used to share information with staff, such as posting QR codes linked to the site's Incident Action Plan at staff locations for easy access to critical site operational and safety information. QR codes were also used as management tools. Site organizers used QR codes to monitor site flow by tracking the amount of time it took vaccine recipients to complete the vaccination process, which was used to provide real-time updates regarding the number of vaccines given, number of individuals queuing, and average wait time.

Prioritizing Risk Management and Quality Control

The sixth theme is associated with techniques that were used to implement redundancies and create fail-safe systems to prevent loss of information and preserve integrity of vaccines. Practices in this theme included using electronic and manual back-up systems for saving information. For example, providers saved the next day's appointment schedule on an alternative system each day, kept paper registration forms as back-ups to electronic systems, and had extra Wi-Fi routers to ensure consistent access to crucial electronic systems (e.g., registration or temperature monitoring). In addition, providers incorporated multiple storage unit temperature checks, despite remote alert mechanisms to prevent temperature excursions. Other quality control items included requiring or encouraging vaccinators to review a vaccinator competency checklist before providing vaccinations and checking vaccine recipient information (e.g., name, date of birth, and vaccine to receive) multiple times throughout the vaccination process to minimize errors.

DISCUSSION

Our findings, drawn from data gathered during early stages of COVID-19 vaccine delivery from vaccination sites across the United States, demonstrated how vaccination providers across the country developed methods to support the timely, safe, and equitable access of COVID-19 vaccines. These site assessments highlighted 6 themes related to promising practices and offer ideas for current and future high-throughput vaccination efforts.

As we have seen historically for seasonal influenza and other vaccines, disparities have been reported in vaccination coverage on the basis of age, race/ethnicity, and location (e.g., rural vs urban settings) throughout the COVID-19 pandemic.[15,16] Although the federal government's initial vaccine rollout plan prioritized equity throughout the vaccination process, health equity was not always considered in COVID-19 vaccine providers' initial vaccine distribution plans.[17] Our findings, however, provide examples of ways that vaccine providers addressed health equity at the vaccination site and worked with partners to improve awareness and vaccine access. These practices, such as partnering with local transit authorities to provide individuals in priority areas free transportation to sites, can be useful for current vaccination providers.

One method to promote health equity at vaccination sites is through strategic partnerships. Previous research has demonstrated the value of strategic and diverse partnerships in public health emergency preparedness for increasing efficiencies and expanding service access.[18–20] Partnerships with trusted community agencies actively working in underresourced communities can be leveraged to successfully conduct outreach. CDC encouraged such partnerships for vaccine outreach in its initial COVID-19 vaccination guidance and is actively working to improve equity in adult immunization across populations disproportionately affected by COVID-19 through partnerships that drive community-level action.[21]

Sufficient and efficiently organized space for recipient flow, vaccine preparation, and communication among staff are important considerations when planning and managing high-throughput vaccination sites.[22] Most of the sites described were considered nontraditional (e.g., sports arenas or convention centers), which likely required more creativity than traditional sites in identifying ways to optimize space and flow for safe and efficient vaccine delivery. Despite having limited experience, site organizers, sometimes with the help of strategic partnerships, attempted to optimize site-specific layout and design to promote process efficiencies and enhance recipient experience.

Visual cues have also been reported to be useful to vaccination sites by, for example, directing individuals to and within a site and efficiently communicating with vaccine recipients and site staff.[23,24] Given the large-scale distribution of novel vaccines from multiple manufacturers with different guidelines, COVID-19 highlighted the importance of clear direction and communication within a vaccination site. QR codes, also used to support efficient communication at vaccination sites, have played a major role in how society shares and collects information since the start of the pandemic, and research has demonstrated the value of QR codes to the health care field and how they are perceived by different groups (e.g., those aged < 70 years may have a higher preference for QR codes).[25–27] Site staff should distribute information based on the needs and preferences of the site's primary users, and findings provide examples of information distribution mechanisms some site organizers have reported as useful.

Beyond QR codes, experts encourage broader use of digital technology for effective and safe delivery of vaccines.[28,29] Scanning 2D barcodes to transfer vaccine data, for example, reduces errors incurred by manual data transfer.[29] Risk management and quality control practices, such as this, improve accuracy and support operations in the event something goes wrong.[30] Manual back-up systems or checks can prevent information loss or errors and can act as secondary safety mechanisms if a malfunction occurs (e.g., power loss or incorrect labeling). Certain processes that might seem redundant or inefficient on a small scale can provide overall operational efficiency during large-scale efforts.[31] Quality assurance standard operating procedures help to ensure successful planning and implementation of risk mitigation and safety protocols.[32] Nevertheless, efficiencies cannot be at the expense of safety. Some assessors observed site staff predrawing syringes and providing them to people administering vaccinations to improve recipient flow. However, according to best practice guidelines, vaccines should be prepared at time of administration because of the potential to introduce errors.[8]

Continuous learning to support improvement of high-throughput vaccination efforts is essential as new approaches might be needed to distribute future vaccine at scale, implement unique storage and handling requirements, or respond to simultaneous outbreaks, such as the COVID-19 pandemic and 2022 mpox outbreak.[33] Shared promising practices can benefit immunization programs and future high-throughput vaccination sites and contribute to continuous improvement of public health emergency activities.

Limitations

The CDC- and FEMA-led assessments were independent efforts with different methodologies, which might have led to variability in promising practices identified. Assessing the strengths and limitations of different assessment methodologies, and the contexts in which they are best suited, could be useful to consider in preparation for possible future pandemics. Although site assessors received training on how to collect promising practice data, variability in data collected among site assessors might have occurred. CDC-led assessments used a train-the-trainer approach to build teams of qualified site assessors. This approach, in which site assessors trained alongside experienced assessors in the field and then went on to train others, helped to rapidly build teams, but might have affected consistency in data collection. Trainers may have inadvertently omitted certain information, or changes or misinterpretation of processes in one trainer may propagate as the train-the-trainer chain continued.

In addition, sites visited were a limited subset of all COVID-19 vaccination sites conducted during the pandemic; these results do not represent all practices developed to enhance efficiency or ability to adhere to guidelines. For example, we likely missed promising practices specific to rural settings because most site assessments occurred in urban areas. Furthermore, these assessments were conducted when vaccines were not yet recommended for anyone younger than 16 years. The practices presented are offered for consideration and might not be appropriate for all sites or situations.

Public Health Implications

The rapid scale-up of COVID-19 vaccination sites was unprecedented and contributed to millions of Americans receiving safe and effective COVID-19 vaccinations.[34] Documenting how sites innovated to improve vaccination operations and implementation is important for future public health emergency responses and high-throughput vaccination efforts. The promising practices identified can be adopted or adapted to potentially increase efficiency and accessibility of current and future high-throughput vaccinations. Further research, such as a recent study by Cho et al.,[35] can be conducted to understand the sustainability, usability, and efficiency of these practices more fully. In the absence of rigorous research, this approach yielded a host of practical measures vaccination providers can consider implementing to enhance operations. AJPH

ABOUT THE AUTHORS

All authors are with the COVID-19 Response's Vaccine Task Force, Centers for Disease Control and Prevention (CDC), Atlanta, GA.

CORRESPONDENCE

Correspondence should be sent to Caitlin McColloch, 1600 Clifton Rd, MS V24-5 Atlanta, GA 30329 (e-mail: oqo4@cdc.gov). Reprints can be ordered at https://ajph.org by clicking the "Reprints" link.

PUBLICATION INFORMATION

Full Citation: McColloch CE, Samson ME, Parris KaeAnne, et al. Promising practices observed in high-throughput COVID-19 vaccination sites in the United States, February–May 2021. *Am J Public Health*. 2023;113(8):909–918.

Acceptance Date: May 1, 2023.

DOI: https://doi.org/10.2105/AJPH.2023.307331

CONTRIBUTORS

All authors made substantial contributions to this article. E. D. Kennedy supervised the project. C. E. McColloch led the development of the article. All authors contributed to the acquisition, analysis, or interpretation of the data and contributed to the drafting or critical revision of the article.

ACKNOWLEDGMENTS

The authors thank all the state and local immunization program management and staff, vaccination site management and staff, Federal Emergency Management Agency (FEMA) Continuous Improvement Program teams, and CDC field staff who helped coordinate and participated in the site assessments described in the article. The authors also thank CDC Site Assessment Team members Glenroy Christie, MPH, Suzanne Friesen, MPP, James Matthias, MPH, Angela Montesanti Porter, MPH, Heidi Pfeiffer, MEd, and Brent Wolff, PhD. Finally, the authors would like to thank Achal Bhatt, PhD, Michelle Banks, MS, Amy Fiebelkorn Parker, MSN, LeAnne Fox, MD, Samuel B. Graitcer, MD, Cameron Noblit, MPH, Janell Routh, MD, Katherine Schwenk, MS-GIST, Sean Trimble, MPH, JoEllen Wolicki, BSN, members of CDC's COVID-19 Response Vaccine Task Force, and the FEMA Continuous Improvement Program for their support and guidance of this work.

Note. The findings and conclusions in this report are those of the authors and do not necessarily represent the official position of the CDC.

CONFLICTS OF INTEREST

The authors declared no potential conflicts of interest with respect to the research, authorship, or publication of this article.

HUMAN PARTICIPANT PROTECTION

This project was determined by CDC to not be human participant research and did not require institutional review board approval. It was conducted consistent with applicable federal law and CDC policy (see, e.g., 45 CFR part 46, 21 CFR part 56; 42 USC §241(d); 5 USC §552a; 44 USC §3501 et seq.).

REFERENCES

1. US Department of Health and Human Services. From the factory to the frontlines: the Operation Warp Speed strategy for distributing a COVID-19 vaccine. 2020. Available at: https://www.hhs.gov/sites/default/files/strategy-for-distributing-covid-19-vaccine.pdf. Accessed May 30, 2023.
2. Rambhia KJ, Watson M, Kirk Sell T, Waldhorn R, Toner E. Mass vaccination for the 2009 H1N1 pandemic: approaches, challenges, and recommendations. *Biosecur Bioterror.* 2010;8(4):321–330. https://doi.org/10.1089/bsp.2010.0043
3. Centers for Disease Control and Prevention. COVID-19 Vaccination Program interim operational guidance jurisdiction operations. US Department of Health and Human Services. 2020. Available at: https://www.cdc.gov/vaccines/imz-managers/downloads/Covid-19-Vaccination-Program-Interim_Playbook.pdf. Accessed May 30, 2023.
4. Goralnick E, Kaufmann C, Gawande A. Mass-vaccination sites—an essential innovation to curb the Covid-19 pandemic. *N Engl J Med.* 2021;384(18):e67. https://doi.org/10.1056/NEJMp2102535
5. Federal Emergency Management Agency. Community Vaccination Centers playbook. 2021. Available at: https://www.fema.gov/disaster/coronavirus/governments/community-vaccination-centers-playbook. Accessed May 30, 2023.
6. Centers for Disease Control and Prevention. How to enroll as a COVID-19 vaccination provider. 2022. Available at: https://www.cdc.gov/vaccines/covid-19/provider-enrollment.html. Accessed April 1, 2022.
7. Centers for Disease Control and Prevention. Interim guidance for routine and influenza immunization services during the COVID-19 pandemic. 2021. Available at: https://www.cdc.gov/vaccines/pandemic-guidance/index.html. Accessed May 30, 2023.
8. Centers for Disease Control and Prevention. Vaccine storage and handling toolkit. 2021. Available at: https://www.cdc.gov/vaccines/hcp/admin/storage/toolkit/storage-handling-toolkit.pdf. Accessed May 30, 2023.
9. Centers for Disease Control and Prevention. COVID-19 vaccine Emergency Use Authorization (EUA) fact sheets for recipients and caregivers. 2021. Available at: https://www.cdc.gov/vaccines/covid-19/eua/index.html. Accessed April 1, 2022.
10. Federal Emergency Management Agency. Continuous Improvement Technical Assistance Program. Available at: https://preptoolkit.fema.gov/web/cip-citap. Accessed April 1, 2022.
11. Centers for Disease Control and Prevention. COVID-19 vaccination reporting systems. 2022. Available at: https://www.cdc.gov/vaccines/covid-19/reporting/overview/IT-systems.html. Accessed April 1, 2022.
12. Centers for Disease Control and Prevention. Vaccines for Children Program (VFC). 2022. Available at: https://www.cdc.gov/vaccines/programs/vfc/index.html. Accessed April 1, 2022.
13. Bingham AJ, Witkowsky P. Deductive and inductive approaches to qualitative data analysis. In: Vanover CMP, Saldana J, eds. *Analyzing and Interpreting Qualitative Research: After the Interview.* Thousand Oaks, CA: SAGE Publications; 2021:133–146.
14. Marmot M, Allen JJ. Social determinants of health equity. *Am J Public Health.* 2014;104(suppl 4):S517–S519. https://doi.org/10.2105/AJPH.2014.302200
15. Kini A, Morgan R, Kuo H, et al. Differences and disparities in seasonal influenza vaccine, acceptance, adverse reactions, and coverage by age, sex, gender, and race. *Vaccine.* 2022;40(11):1643–1654. https://doi.org/10.1016/j.vaccine.2021.04.013
16. Saelee R, Zell E, Murthy BP, et al. Disparities in COVID-19 vaccination coverage between urban and rural counties—United States, December 14, 2020–January 31, 2022. *MMWR Morb Mortal Wkly Rep.* 2022;71(9):335–340. https://doi.org/10.15585/mmwr.mm7109a2
17. Hardeman A, Wong T, Denson JL, Postelnicu R, Rojas JC. Evaluation of health equity in COVID-19 vaccine distribution plans in the United States. *JAMA Netw Open.* 2021;4(7):e2115653. https://doi.org/10.1001/jamanetworkopen.2021.15653
18. Findley SE, Irigoyen M, See D, et al. Community–provider partnerships to reduce immunization disparities: field report from northern Manhattan. *Am J Public Health.* 2003;93(7):1041–1044. https://doi.org/10.2105/AJPH.93.7.1041
19. Erwin PC, Parks RG, Mazzucca S, et al. Evidence-based public health provided through local health departments: importance of academic–practice partnerships. *Am J Public Health.* 2019;109(5):739–747. https://doi.org/10.2105/AJPH.2019.304958
20. Viera AJ, Barnett J, Case M, et al. Partnerships to care for our patients and communities during COVID-19. *J Am Board Fam Med.* 2021;34(5):1003–1009. https://doi.org/10.3122/jabfm.2021.05.210091
21. Centers for Disease Control and Prevention. A guide for community partners: increasing COVID-19 vaccine uptake among members of racial and ethnic minority communities. 2021. Available at: https://www.cdc.gov/vaccines/covid-19/downloads/guide-community-partners.pdf. Accessed May 30, 2023.
22. Goldbert SA, Callaway D, Resnick-Ault D, et al. Critical concepts for COVID-19 mass vaccination site operations. *Disaster Med Public Health Prep.* 2021:17:e60. https://doi.org/10.1017/dmp.2021.319
23. Centers for Disease Control and Prevention. Receiving, distributing, and dispensing strategic national stockpile assets: a guide for preparedness, version 11. 2014. Available at: https://www.hsdl.org/c/abstract/?docid=799144. Accessed May 30, 2023.
24. Swift MD, Aliyu MH, Byrne DW, et al. Emergency preparedness in the workplace: the flulapalooza model for mass vaccination. *Am J Public Health.* 2017;107(suppl 2):S168–S176. https://doi.org/10.2105/AJPH.2017.303953
25. Wahsheh HAM, Al-Zahrani MS. Secure and usable QR codes for healthcare systems: the case of COVID-19 pandemic. In: *12th International Conference on Information and Communication Systems.* Valencia, Spain: Institute of Electrical or Electronics Engineers; 2021:324–329. https://doi.org/10.1109/ICICS52457.2021.9464565
26. Sharara S, Radia S. Quick response (QR) codes for patient information delivery: a digital innovation during the coronavirus pandemic. *J Orthod.* 2022;49(1):89–97. https://doi.org/10.1177/14653125211031568
27. Azad A, Alistair D, Laidlaw H, Orlans HO. Using QR smartphone technology to improve patient communication and information distribution. *Eye (Lond).* 2022;36(6):1321–1322. https://doi.org/10.1038/s41433-021-01757-x
28. Lachman P, van der Wilden E. Use of barcode technology can make a difference to patient safety in the post-COVID era. *IJQHC Communications.* 2021;1(1):lyab014. https://doi.org/10.1093/ijcoms/lyab014
29. Reed JH, Evanson HV, Cox R, et al. Improving utilization of vaccine two-dimensional (2D) barcode

scanning technology maximizes accuracy benefits. *J Healthc Qual*. 2021;43(1):39–47. https://doi.org/10.1097/JHQ.0000000000000265

30. Tocco Tussardi I, Tardivo S. Improving risk management by learning from adverse events: report on one year of COVID-19 vaccination campaign in Verona (Northeastern Italy). *Int J Environ Res Public Health*. 2022;19(6):3635. https://doi.org/10.3390/ijerph19063635
31. Tay HL. Lean improvement practices: lessons from healthcare service delivery chains. *IFAC-PapersOnLine*. 2016;49(12):1158–1163. https://doi.org/10.1016/j.ifacol.2016.07.660
32. McKibben LJ, Strange PV, Sneller V, Strikas RA, Rodewald LE. Use of standing orders programs to increase adult vaccination rates: recommendations of the Advisory Committee on Immunization Practices. *MMWR Recomm Rep*. 2000;49(RR-1):15–16.
33. Palmore TN, Henderson DK. Adding new fuel to the fire: monkeypox in the time of COVID-19—implications for health care personnel. *Ann Intern Med*. 2022;175(8):1183–1184. https://doi.org/10.7326/M22-1763
34. Suthar AB. Public health impact of COVID-19 vaccines in the US: observational study. *BMJ*. 2022;337:e069317. https://doi.org/10.1136/bmj-2021-069317
35. Cho B, Athar HM, Bates LG, et al. Patient flow time data of COVID-19 vaccination clinics in 23 sites, United States, April and May 2021. *SSRN*. August 6, 2022. https://doi.org/10.1016/j.vaccine.2022.12.013

Erratum In: "'Ashamed to Put My Name to It': Monsanto, Industrial Bio-Test Laboratories, and the Use of Fraudulent Science, 1969–1985"

In: Rosner D, Markowitz G. "Ashamed to put my name to it": Monsanto, Industrial Bio-Test Laboratories, and the use of fraudulent science, 1969–1985. *Am J Public Health*. 2023;113(6):661–666.

When originally published, the title of the article was listed incorrectly. On p. 661, the title should read: "'Ashamed' to Put His Name to It: Monsanto, Industrial Bio-Test Laboratories, and the Use of Fraudulent Science, 1969–1985."

This change does not affect the article's conclusions. AJPH

https://doi.org/10.2105/AJPH.2023.307247e

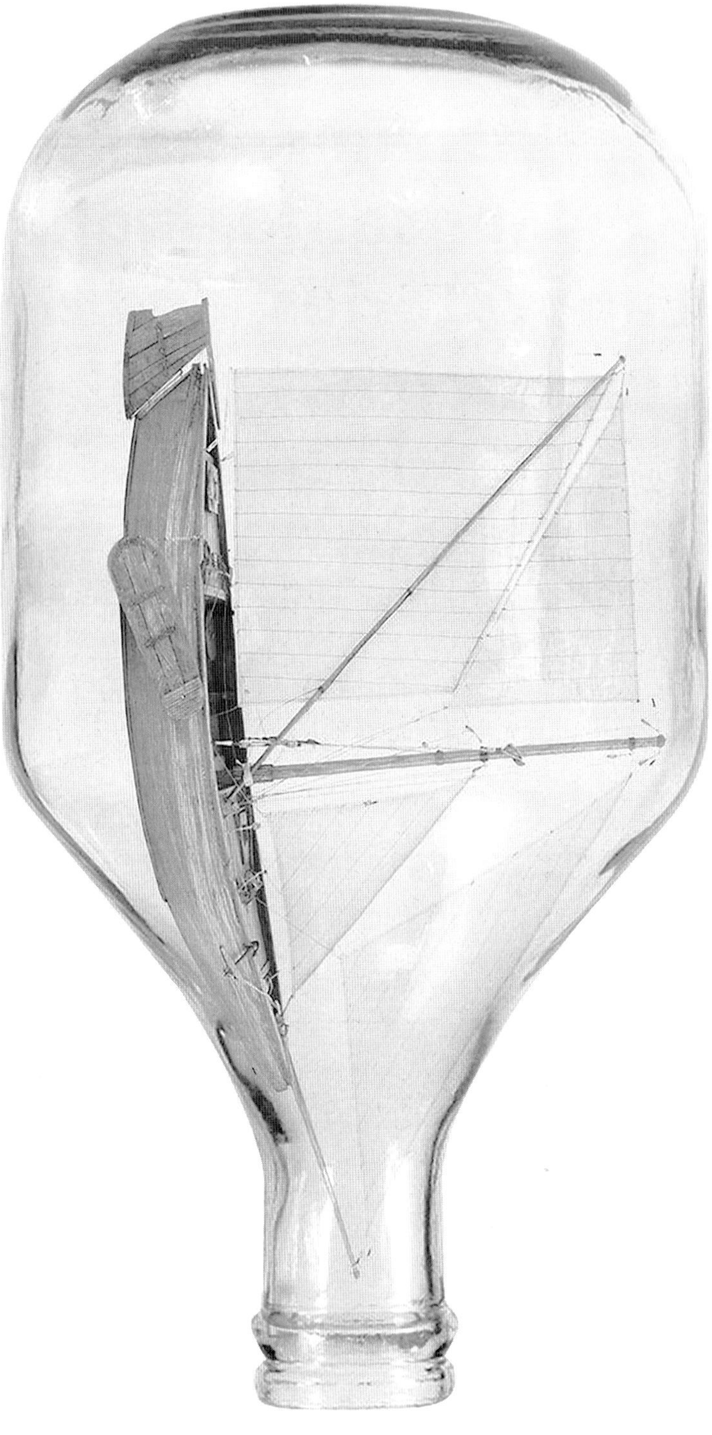

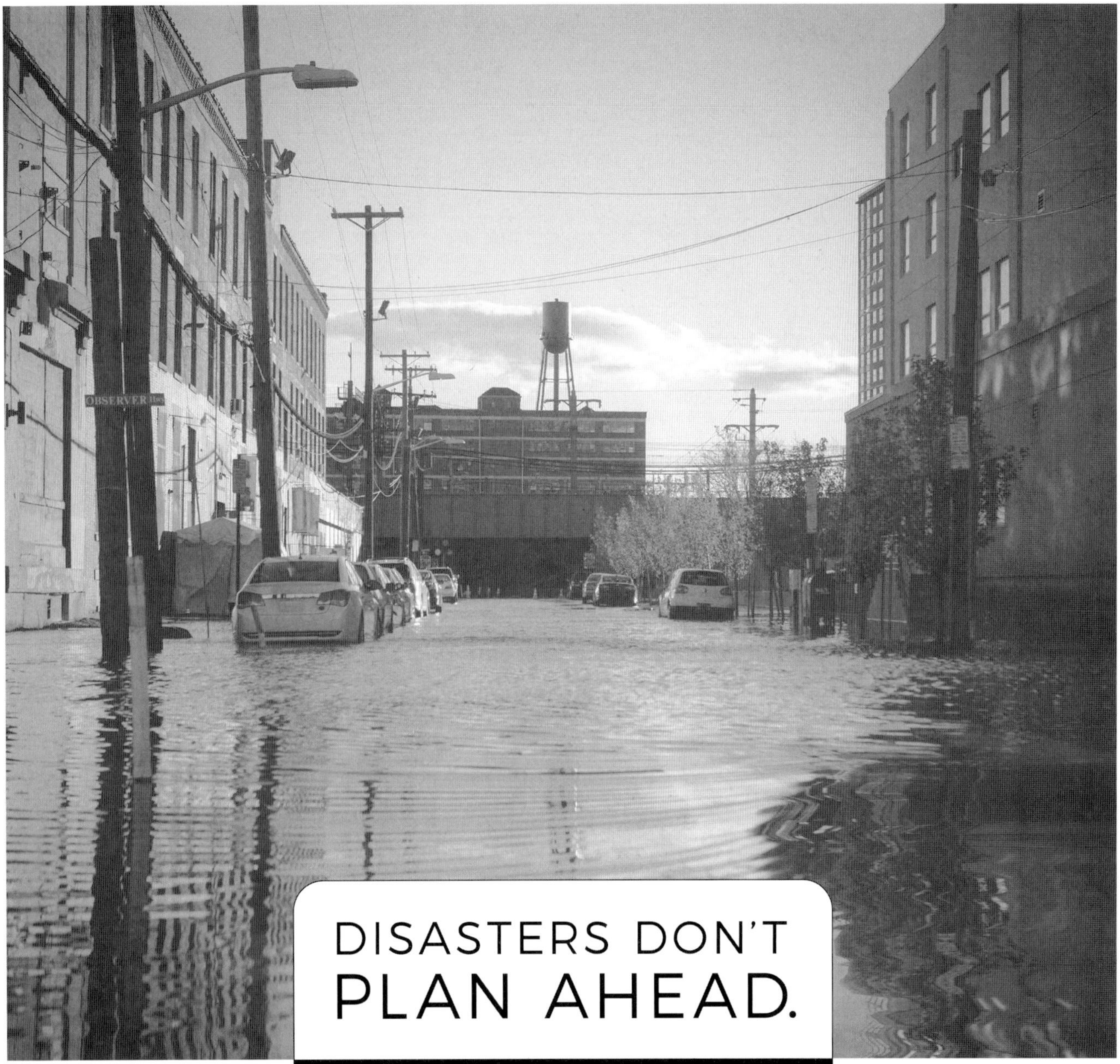

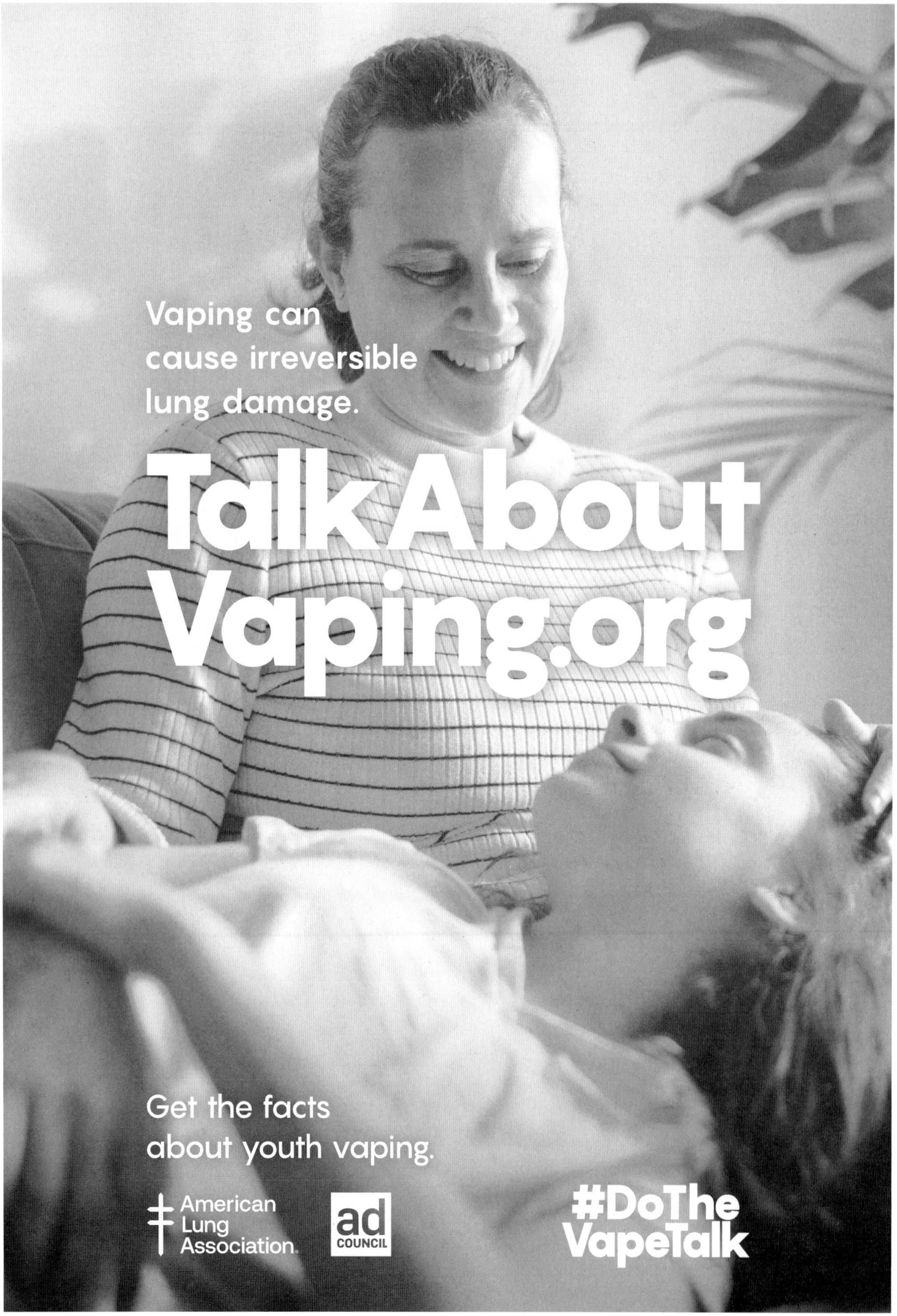

Vaping can cause irreversible lung damage.
TalkAboutVaping.org
Get the facts about youth vaping.
American Lung Association
ad COUNCIL
#DoTheVapeTalk

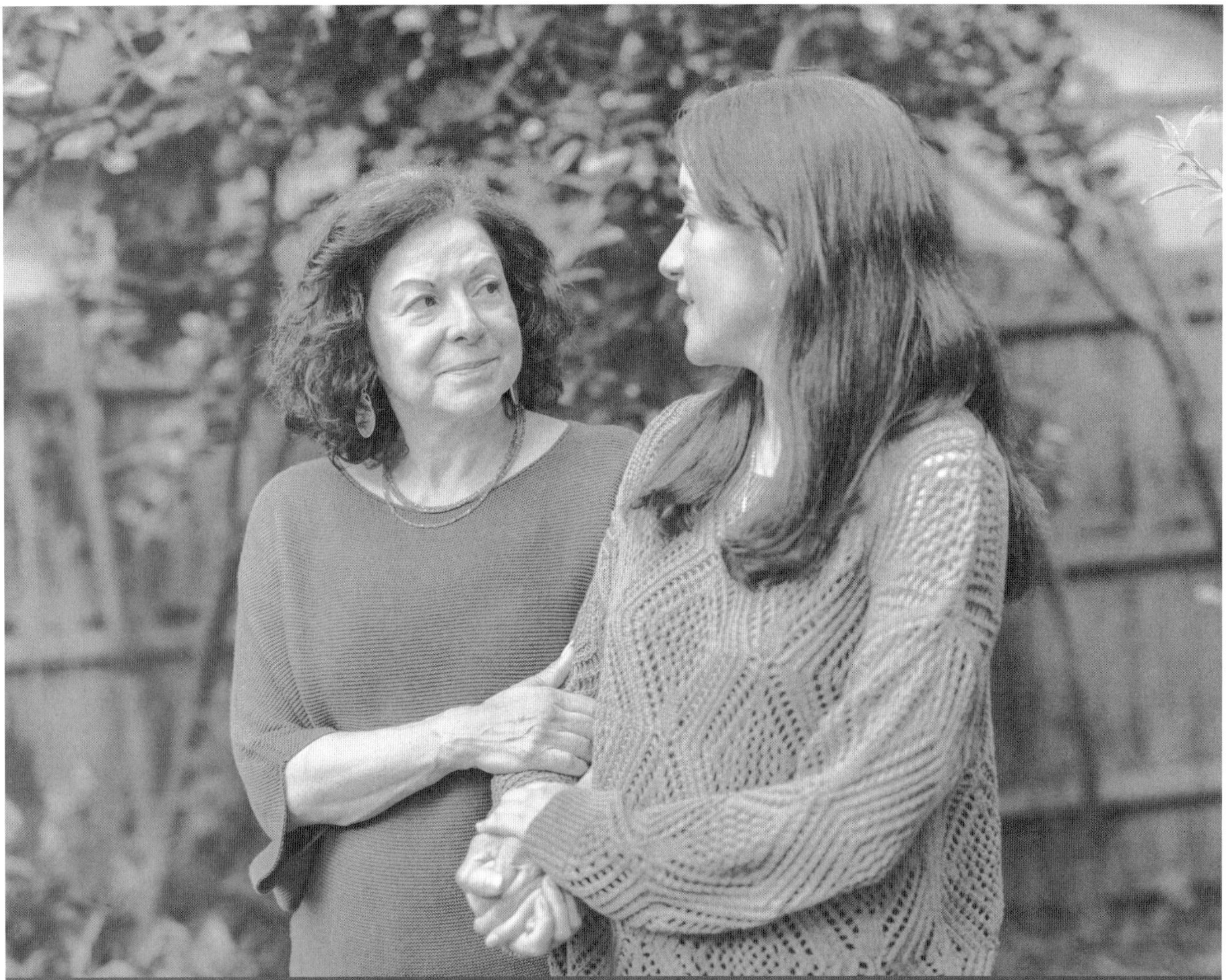

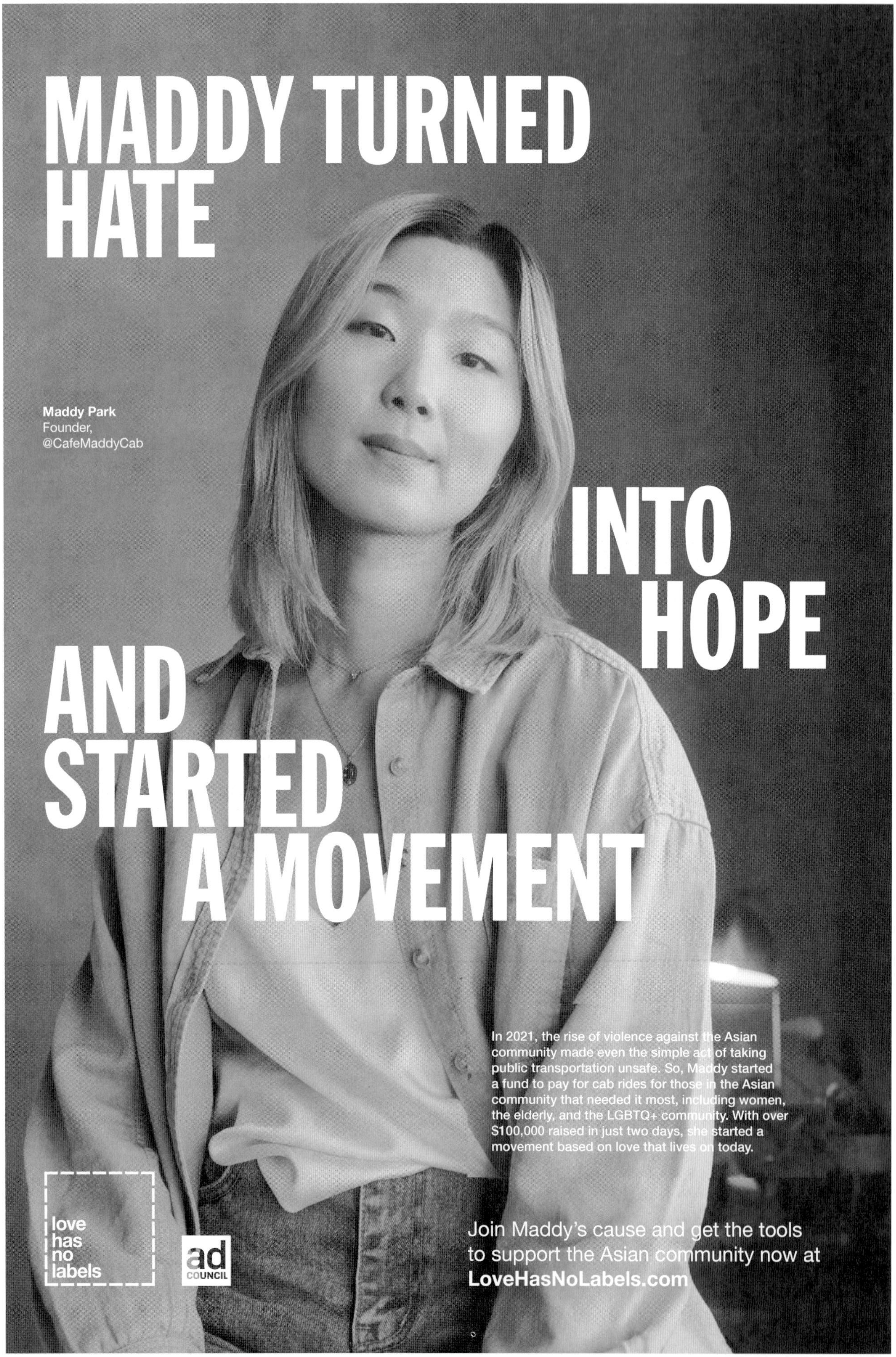
MADDY TURNED HATE
Maddy Park
Founder,
@CafeMaddyCab
INTO HOPE
AND STARTED A MOVEMENT
In 2021, the rise of violence against the Asian community made even the simple act of taking public transportation unsafe. So, Maddy started a fund to pay for cab rides for those in the Asian community that needed it most, including women, the elderly, and the LGBTQ+ community. With over $100,000 raised in just two days, she started a movement based on love that lives on today.
love has no labels
ad COUNCIL
Join Maddy's cause and get the tools to support the Asian community now at
LoveHasNoLabels.com

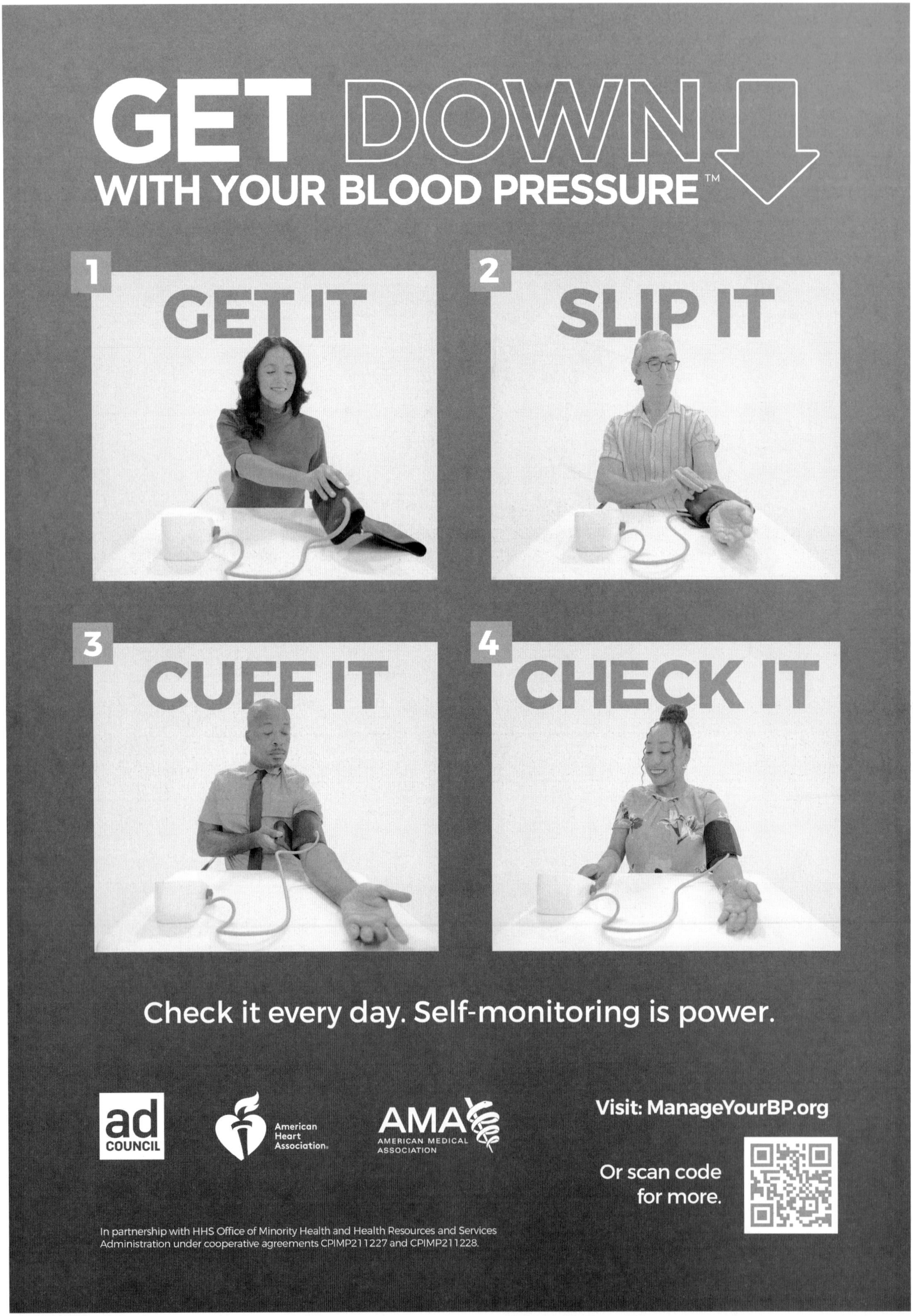
GET DOWN
WITH YOUR BLOOD PRESSURE™
1
GET IT
2
SLIP IT
3
CUFF IT
4
CHECK IT
Check it every day. Self-monitoring is power.
ad COUNCIL
American Heart Association.
AMA AMERICAN MEDICAL ASSOCIATION
Visit: ManageYourBP.org
Or scan code for more.
In partnership with HHS Office of Minority Health and Health Resources and Services Administration under cooperative agreements CPIMP211227 and CPIMP211228.